Case Presentations in Re

Case Presentations in Respiratory Medicine

John A. Elliott, BSc, MB, ChB, FRCP(Glas.)
Consultant Physician, Heathfield Hospital, Ayr
Honorary Clinical Lecturer, University of Glasgow

Butterworths
London   Boston   Singapore   Sydney   Toronto   Wellington

PART OF REED INTERNATIONAL P.L.C.

First published 1989

© Butterworth & Co. (Publishers) Ltd, 1989

British Library Cataloguing in Publication Data

Elliott, John A (John Arthur)
    Case presentations in respiratory medicine.
    1. Man. Respiratory system. Diagnosis &
    therapy
    I. title
    616.2

    ISBN 0-407-00810-1

British Library Cataloging-in-Publication Data

Elliott, John A.
    Case presentations in respiratory medicine / John A. Elliott.
        p. cm.
    Includes index.
    ISBN 0-407-00810-1
    1. Respiratory organs--Diseases--Case studies. 2. Respiratory
organs--Diseases--Examinations, questions, etc. I. Title.
    [DNLM: 1. Respiratory Tract Diseases--case studies.
2. Respiratory Tract Diseases--examination questions.   WF 18 E46c]
RC732.E45 1989
616.2'09--dc19
DNLM/DLC   88-36739

Photoset by Butterworths Litho Preparation Department
Printed and bound in Great Britain by Butler and Tanner, Frome, Somerset

Preface

The specialty of respiratory medicine has undergone great changes in recent decades. The tuberculosis era has been replaced by an epidemic of smoking-related disorders, but the burden of disease remains considerable. In the UK respiratory disorders, including lung cancer, are second only to cardiac disease as the leading cause of death. Respiratory illness causes by far the greatest number of days lost from work and the largest number of visits to a general practitioner. The advent of fibreoptic bronchoscopy and other new diagnostic techniques, advances in our understanding of the pathogenesis of respiratory disorders, the appearance of new diseases, new treatments and fresh therapeutic challenges render respiratory medicine as relevant to the modern clinician as it was to our nineteenth century colleagues.

In common with other texts in Butterworth's Case Presentations series this book is intended primarily as a revision aid for postgraduates sitting higher examinations. It is also aimed at the wider audience of all practising physicians who see patients with lung disease and who seek to update their knowledge in as painless a way as possible in this changing field.

The case histories (names have been changed in order to preserve confidentiality) forming the first part of the book are each followed by questions which test diagnostic ability and competence in the planning of further investigations and clinical management. The cases have been selected to encompass a broad range of subjects. All have been encountered in clinical practice over a period of three years in a district hospital setting and, although some rarities are included, the emphasis is on common problems, pitfalls and recent developments. The second part of the book is an answer section where each diagnosis is treated to a brief clinical review. In most cases key references have been appended to the text for those wishing to pursue a particular issue in greater depth.

Look at this book as a series of 'talking points in respiratory medicine'. It cannot compete with the detail offered in standard textbooks, but I trust that it offers to the reader the opportunity of discovering some aspects of this fascinating specialty in a more realistic and entertaining fashion than is possible with more demanding and comprehensive but, possibly, less stimulating works.

John A. Elliott

Acknowledgements

My gratitude is due to those medical students and postgraduates for whom this book was written. Without their interest and enthusiasm the project would never have been conceived. I owe my thanks to friends and colleagues for contributing some of the clinical material upon which the book is based and I owe a special debt to Dr Neil Thomson of the Western Infirmary, Glasgow for his encouragement and constructive comments on the text. I am particularly grateful to Ms Valerie Preston for her skilful production of the illustrations. Last, but not least, I thank my wife Jackie for her support and forebearance at all stages of the book's preparation.

Contents

Abbreviations, terms and units

FEV_1	Forced expiratory volume in 1 second (litre)
VC	Vital capacity (litre)
FVC	Forced vital capacity (litre)
FRC	Functional residual capacity (litre)
RV	Residual volume (litre)
TLC	Total lung capacity (litre)
PEFR	Peak expiratory flow rate (l/min)
V_A	Volume of alveolar gas (litre)
TL_{co}	Total carbon monoxide gas transfer capacity (mmol/ min per kPa)
K_{co}	Carbon monoxide gas transfer coefficient (mmol/min per kPa per litre)
Pa_{O_2}	Partial pressure of oxygen in arterial blood (kPa)
Pa_{CO_2}	Partial pressure of carbon dioxide in arterial blood (kPa)
FI_{O_2}	Fraction of oxygen in inspired air

Case Presentations and Questions

Case 1 ✓

Mr Robert Thomson, a 63-year-old shipyard worker, was referred to medical outpatients with a history of persistent cough and increased breathlessness on exertion of four weeks duration. Over the same period he had lost about seven pounds in weight. In retrospect he had been aware of shortness of breath when climbing hills for some years, but he had put this down to his age. He admitted to wheeze on an occasional basis but recently this had been no more evident than usual. He was an ex-smoker of nine years duration but, prior to this, he had smoked 20 cigarettes daily since the age of 18.

For some months Mr Thomson had suffered central chest 'tightness' when walking out, especially on cold mornings. He

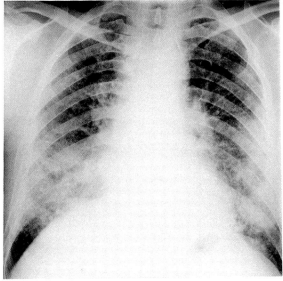

Figure Q1.1

1

denied any episodes of prolonged chest pain and gave no history of nocturnal dyspnoea or ankle swelling. One of Mr Thomson's two brothers had died from a myocardial infarct at the age of 56 and another, younger brother, suffered from angina.

Physical examination revealed no evidence of finger clubbing. Mr Thomson was afebrile with a regular cardiac rhythm at a rate of 78 beats/min, blood pressure 138/80. Heart sounds and jugular venous pressure were normal. Scattered wheezes were audible throughout both lung fields, with no other adventitious sounds. There were no abnormal abdominal findings but rectal examination revealed an enlarged irregular prostate. The haemoglobin was 15.7 g/dl, white blood count 10.1×10^9/l, ESR 36 mm/h. The ECG was normal and the chest X-ray (Figure Q1.1) was reported as showing bilateral diffuse intrapulmonary shadowing, right basal pleural thickening and right-sided diaphragmatic calcification. Bronchoscopy showed no visible abnormality. Lung function tests gave the results shown in Table Q1.1

Table Q1.1 Results of lung function tests*

	Predicted	Actual	% Predicted
FEV_1	3.00	1.95	65.0
FVC	4.14	2.90	70.0
FEV/FVC%	68.6	67.2	100.0
RV	2.30	1.77	77.0
TLC	6.50	4.52	69.5
TL_{co}	8.99	6.81	75.8

* For abbreviations and units, see page x.

Questions

1. Describe the abnormality of pulmonary function.
2. Suggest a clinical differential diagnosis.
3. What further respiratory investigations would you consider?

Case 2

A 44-year-old unemployed ex-merchant seaman, Mr Laurence Albert, was admitted to the medical unit after suffering several episodes of brisk haemoptysis over a period of about two hours. The patient estimated that he had produced approximately half a pint of fresh blood. He gave no prior history of haemoptysis and indicated no recent change in his longstanding smoker's cough productive of mucoid sputum. There was no history of chest pain, breathlessness or wheeze but Mr Albert did admit to a poor appetite and in the previous three months he had lost about seven pounds in weight.

Ten years before Mr Albert had undergone vagotomy and gastroenterostomy for chronic duodenal ulcer. At around this time, and for some years before, he admitted to a regular and heavy intake of alcohol and he had received counselling for alcoholism. Subsequently, he had remained susceptible to frequent alcoholic binges, but at the time of admission he claimed to have been 'dry' for some months. He had smoked 20 cigarettes a day for 20 years.

On admission Mr Albert was still producing small quantities of fresh blood. He was afebrile but appeared anxious and had a tachycardia of 110 beats/min. Physical examination revealed nicotine-stained fingers. Auscultation of the chest disclosed early

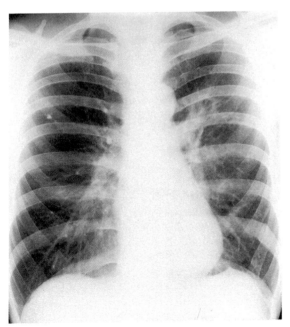

Figure Q2.1

inspiratory crackles in both lung fields, predominantly at the left lung base. Abdominal examination was normal.

The haemoglobin was 11.2 g/dl with a normochromic normocytic blood film. The white blood count was $6.6 \times 10^9/l$. The chest X-ray (Figure Q2.1) showed an ill-defined shadow adjacent to the upper pole of the left hilum, a small right mid-zone shadow of calcific density and calcification of the right hilum. The patient's heavily bloodstained sputum showed moderate numbers of pus cells on microscopy but repeated specimens were negative on direct smear (Ziehl-Neelsen stain) for acid-alcohol fast bacilli. Initial sputum cultures yielded no significant pathogens. A tuberculin test was positive to ten tuberculin units (0.1 ml of 1/1000 old tuberculin), with 30 mm of induration. During fibreoptic bronchoscopy, some days after his admission, altered blood was noted throughout the left bronchial tree but there was no other specific abnormality. Bronchial aspirate was negative for malignant cells and two days later, cultures were sterile.

Questions

1. What is the probable diagnosis?
2. Give two alternative diagnoses that should be considered.

Case 3

Mrs Angela Warren, a 52-year-old housewife, was referred to the chest clinic in May, 1984, after a prolonged period of ill health. Over the previous seven months she had felt generally unwell, anorexic and had lost about a stone in weight. Over this same period she had felt intermittently feverish and had suffered a persistent cough, regularly productive of variable quantities of purulent sputum, as well as occasional haemoptysis. Repeated short courses of antibiotic had, on each occasion, produced only a temporary amelioration of her symptoms. Earlier, for some years, she had been prone to episodes of bronchitis during the winter months but for the most part her usual smoker's cough had been unproductive of sputum. She had smoked 20–30 cigarettes a day for 30 years.

Mrs Warren had attended medical outpatients on two previous occasions. In 1977 her general practitioner had asked for advice regarding the patient's complaint that her 'heart was always racing'. An anxiety state was diagnosed. In June 1983, she was referred again with a six month history of lethargy and breathlessness. The latter symptom was accompanied by frequent sighing and the sensation of being unable to completely fill her lungs. Chest and abdominal examination revealed no abnormality at this time, a chest X-ray was reported as normal and spirometric values were within normal limits. She was reassured and discharged from the clinic. The only other relevant medical history was a surgical admission in September, 1983, when Mrs Warren underwent an emergency laparotomy for a perforated duodenal ulcer. Postoperatively, she made good progress except for an abdominal sinus which discharged purulent material for some weeks before eventually healing up.

When seen in the chest clinic Mrs Warren appeared anxious and readily confessed to her fear that she had cancer. There was a fine tremor of the outstretched hands, a tachycardia of 110 beats/min and a low grade pyrexia of 37.4°C. Definite finger clubbing was noted. Examination of the chest revealed a reduction in breath sounds at both bases as well as bi-basal, early inspiratory crackles. Abdominal examination revealed a well healed laparotomy scar and a smooth, slightly tender, epigastric mass. The haemoglobin was 10.6 g/dl; red cell indices were abnormally reduced (MCV 72 fl, HCt 0.347, MCH 24.1PG) but the blood film showed only mild anisocytosis. The white blood count was $10.9 \times 10^9/l$ (84% neutrophils), ESR 72 mm/h. A chest radiograph was reported as showing ill-defined right basal consolidation. The patient's mucopurulent sputum yielded no significant growth. Fibreoptic bronchoscopy showed localized inflammatory changes involving the right middle and lower lobe bronchi. The bronchial aspirate was sterile and cytology was negative for malignant cells.

Questions

1. What is the most likely diagnosis?
2. Suggest two imaging procedures for confirming this diagnosis.

Case 4

A 19-year-old labourer was admitted to the medical unit with a history of left pleuritic chest pain and severe breathlessness of sudden onset. He was too distressed to give a detailed medical history but, after treatment, he admitted to a non-productive cough and shortness of breath on exertion which had progressed in severity over a period of three years. He was a keen footballer but had found that for the previous 12 months he had been unable to complete a game because he tired easily; he confessed to having to stop after climbing just three flights of stairs. He had smoked 15 cigarettes a day for two years.

As a child he had been followed at a paediatric hospital from the age of two until he was 12 years old because of a cardiac systolic murmur. When aged four he had undergone cardiac catheterization which confirmed the presence of a small ventricular septal defect, with a 5% step-up in oxygen saturation in the right ventricle. He had been asymptomatic during this period and a chest radiograph taken just prior to his discharge from the paediatric unit was reported as normal. There was no family history of respiratory disease.

On admission to the medical unit, examination revealed signs consistent with a left-sided tension pneumothorax and this diagnosis was confirmed on a portable chest X-ray. Insertion of an intercostal tube with an underwater seal led to reinflation of the lung and there was no recurrence of the pneumothorax when the drain was removed three days later. A more thorough physical examination of the chest, than had been possible initially, showed a generalized reduction in breath sounds throughout both lung

Table Q4.1   Results of pulmonary function tests*

	Predicted	Actual	% Predicted
FEV$_1$	4.08	1.47	36.0
FVC	4.93	3.01	61.1
FEV/FVC%	78.6	48.8	62.1
RV	1.56	3.13	200.6
TLC	6.08	6.14	101.1
TL_{co}	10.65	5.86	55.0
K_{co}	1.88	1.50	79.8

* For abbreviations and units, see page x.

fields, but there were no adventitious sounds. There was a pansystolic murmur loudest at the left sternal edge. A repeat chest radiograph, taken in the X-ray department, and therefore of superior quality to the original portable film, showed a bilateral diffuse intrapulmonary abnormality consisting of a remarkably uniform pattern of honeycomb shadows. Routine haematological and biochemical values were normal as were serum levels of angiotensin converting enzyme and α_1-antitrypsin. Pulmonary function tests gave the results shown in Table Q4.1.

Questions

1. What is the most likely diagnosis?
2. Suggest three relevant investigations.

Case 5

A 40-year-old housewife was referred for a specialist opinion after a chest infection had apparently failed to resolve. Three months earlier she had suffered an influenza-like illness and following this she had developed a cough productive of mucopurulent sputum. There was no history of chest pain, haemoptysis or shortness of breath, but she had been aware of a tendency to wheeze. Her cough had persisted and remained troublesome for some weeks with no clear response to antibiotic therapy. By the time of her clinic attendence, however, her cough had virtually resolved although she continued to complain of wheeze.

Eight years before, the patient had suffered a similar illness in association with left-sided 'pleurisy' and since this time she had been aware of occasional wheezing, especially at times of upper respiratory infection. There was no history of childhood asthma and the patient was a lifelong non-smoker.

Physical examination revealed noisy inspiratory breath sounds audible at the mouth, impairment of the percussion note and a fixed monophonic wheeze at the left base. Lung function tests showed normal spirometry and peak expiratory flow rate; static

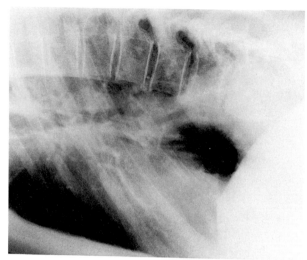

Figure Q5.2

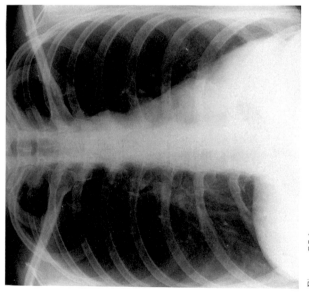

Figure Q5.1

lung volumes were at the lower limits of normal. The patient's postero-anterior and left lateral chest radiographs are illustrated in Figures Q5.1 and Q5.2, respectively.

Questions

1. What is the most likely diagnosis?
2. Suggest two further relevant investigations at this stage.

Case 6

Mrs Roselyn Barrie, a 70-year-old former secretary, was referred to medical outpatients with a seven month history of unproductive cough and progressive exertional dyspnoea. She denied any gastrointestinal or genitourinary symptomatology but systematic enquiry did reveal a history of infrequent angina of effort of several years' duration. Twelve years before she had undergone a successful pelvic floor repair and at the age of 37 she underwent a partial thyroidectomy for thyrotoxicosis. Mrs Barrie had been a lifelong non-smoker and she rarely drank alcohol. Her medication had remained unchanged for ten years and consisted of acebutolol in standard dosage and the occasional use of sublingual glyceryl trinitrate.

Mrs Barrie appeared fit for her age. In the chest, physical signs suggested the presence of pleural fluid at the right base. The jugular venous pressure was normal and there was no dependent oedema. Abdominal examination revealed a large, firm, smooth, non-tender mass apparently arising from the pelvis. There was no clinical evidence of ascites or hepatomegaly.

Routine haematology and biochemical tests, including thyroid function, were normal. A chest radiograph confirmed the presence of a moderate right pleural effusion and, following pleural aspiration, a repeat film showed clear lung fields. The heart size and silhouette were normal. The pleural fluid proved to be a sterile, straw-coloured exudate (protein 35 g/l). Cytological examination showed reactive mesothelial cells only. Multiple pleural biopsies showed no evidence of malignancy. An abdominal ultrasound demonstrated some ascitic fluid and showed a large, well defined, solid mass (?ovarian) lying above the bladder.

Questions

1. What is the probable diagnosis?
2. Are any further tests required?

Case 7

Mr James Peterson, a 31-year-old long distance coach driver, had never taken his health seriously. He was grossly overweight, smoked 60 cigarettes a day and until the day of his admission to hospital he claimed that he had never consulted a doctor. For six weeks he had been off his food and, latterly, anorexia had been accompanied by nausea, retching and occasional vomiting. For four weeks he had become progressively more lethargic with breathlessness, also a new feature, noticeable on moderate exertion. He was finally encouraged to see his general practitioner after he developed intermittent haemoptysis, but only after this had persisted for six days. His general practitioner arranged hospital admission later the same day after the surgery had been phoned with the results of Mr Peterson's laboratory investigations.

Systematic enquiry later revealed a history of intermittent haemoptysis over a period of 18 months. Mr Peterson had not been unduly worried by this, claiming that the symptom settled if he stopped smoking for a few days! There was no history of abdominal pain and he denied any genitourinary symptomatology except, perhaps, for a recent tendency to pass rather less urine than usual. There was no relevant past medical history and he was taking no medication.

On examination he was grossly obese and clinically anaemic. The pulse rate was 92 beats/min, blood pressure 180/96 and there was a soft systolic ejection murmur heard maximally at the left sternal edge. There was no evidence of retinopathy, the venous pressure was normal, there was no peripheral oedema and the chest was clear on auscultation. The haemoglobin was 4.4 g/dl, the blood film showing slight hypochromia and moderate anisocytosis with some rod forms and a few burr cells. The blood urea was 74.7 mmol/l and the serum creatinine was an almost incredible 4215 μmol/l. Urine microscopy showed moderate numbers of red cells and white cells as well as scanty granular casts. An ECG was normal. The chest film was reported as showing bilateral ill-defined alveolar consolidation. Lung function tests showed a restrictive ventilatory defect with a raised K_{co} (corrected for blood haemoglobin).

Questions

1. What is the most likely diagnosis?
2. Suggest two further *specific* investigations.

Case 8

Mr Robert Pantling, a 48-year-old pipe lagger, had spent most of his working days in the Glasgow shipyards. Despite having been a smoker of 30 cigarettes a day he had enjoyed good health and, apart from a previous knee cartilage operation many years before, there was no relevant past medical history. A chest clinic appointment was secured, however, when Mr Pantling saw his general practitioner with a complaint of breathlessness on exertion. There had been a subacute onset, with the severity of dyspnoea increasing over several days to the point where he had felt unable to continue at work.

When first seen in the chest clinic there were both clinical and radiological signs of a moderate left pleural effusion. Mr Pantling confessed to a longstanding smoker's cough. There was a family history of rheumatoid arthritis but the patient himself denied joint symptoms and his serum was negative for rheumatoid factor. Pleural aspiration yielded a straw-coloured exudate containing predominantly lymphocytes; no malignant cells were seen and cultures (including those for tubercle bacilli) were uniformly negative. After the effusion had been aspirated to dryness a repeat chest film showed no specific abnormality and bronchoscopy was normal.

In the absence of a definite diagnosis Mr Pantling was treated for tuberculosis but, despite this, the effusion recurred and, six months following his initial presentation, a left thoracotomy and decortication was carried out. At operation there was evidence of marked fibrous pleural thickening and histological examination of the resected material showed chronically inflamed and fibrotic pleura with no evidence of tuberculosis or malignancy. He remained well, with breathlessness noticeable only on moderately severe exertion, until 18 months later when he developed a moderate right pleural effusion. Once again examination of pleural fluid failed to suggest a specific diagnosis. He subsequently underwent a right decortication when the operative findings were similar to those which had been recorded on the left side two years earlier.

When seen two years after his second operation he was well but breathless on moderate exertion. His chest X-ray showed diffuse bilateral pleural thickening. Lung function tests showed mild restriction of lung volumes and a raised K_{co}.

Questions

1. What is the probable diagnosis?
2. Are there any medicolegal implications?
3. Name two other pleural/pulmonary conditions from which Mr Pantling remains at increased risk.

Case 9

Mr Joel Benjamin, a 30-year-old West Indian immigrant, consulted his general practitioner with a three weeks' history of joint pain which, first of all, had been localized to the left elbow but which subsequently affected the wrists, proximal interphalangeal joints of both hands and both knees and ankles. Just prior to the onset of symptoms he had suffered a severe sore throat. An anti-streptolysin O titre gave no evidence of recent streptococcal infection and serum was negative for rheumatoid factor. A tentative diagnosis of 'reactive arthritis' was made and the patient was prescribed a non-steroidal anti-inflammatory drug.

Specialist referral followed when, over a period of three months, he continued to suffer joint pain, felt intermittently feverish and lost about half a stone in weight. When seen later in medical outpatients he denied any respiratory symptomatology except for a dry cough of recent onset. Mr Benjamin was a lifelong non-smoker.

On examination he was mildly pyrexial (37.5°C). There was no evidence of finger clubbing or synovitis. Small scattered nodular skin infiltrations were noted over the patient's trunk. Chest auscultation revealed no adventitious sounds. The haemoglobin was 13.4 g/dl, white blood count 6.9 × 10^9/l, ESR 30 mm/h. Total plasma globulins were markedly elevated at 53 g/l, the electrophoretic strip showing a predominant increase in gammaglobulin and a smaller increase in α_2-globulin. Rheumatoid factor was now positive at a titre of 1/320. Liver function tests showed slightly elevated serum transaminases. A tuberculin test (dilution: 1/1000) gave no induration. The chest radiograph showed extensive bilateral shadowing in the middle and lower zones, partly obscuring the lung hila. Radiographs of the hands, knees and feet were normal. Pulmonary function tests showed minor restriction of lung volumes and normal gas transfer.

Questions

1. What is the most likely diagnosis?
2. How might the diagnosis be most readily confirmed in this case?

Case 10

Miss Jane Fields, a 73-year-old retired secretary, was referred for further investigation following an episode of 'pneumonia' which had apparently failed to resolve. She had first presented to her general practitioner with a four week history of cough productive of mucoid sputum. Focal chest signs were noted in the left lower zone posteriorly and a chest film, arranged by the general practitioner, showed homogeneous consolidation affecting the left lower lobe. Despite combined treatment with amoxycillin and erythromycin her symptoms and signs failed to improve. Clinic referral was arranged when a repeat chest X-ray, taken three weeks after her initial presentation, showed more extensive left lower lobe consolidation.

When seen in the chest clinic, physical examination revealed no abnormal physical signs apart from an impaired percussion note and late inspiratory crackles at the left lung base posteriorly. There was no prior history of respiratory symptomatology and Miss Fields had been a lifelong non-smoker. The haemoglobin was 13.6 g/dl, white blood count $6.3 \times 10^9/l$ with a normal differential, ESR 16 mm/h. The patient's mucoid sputum yielded no pathogens on either routine or, subsequently, tuberculous culture and repeated specimens were negative for malignant cells. Fibreoptic bronchoscopy showed no definite abnormality. No further investigations were undertaken at this stage.

When seen three months later, however, there had been a clear deterioration. Miss Field's cough had become more distressing and increasingly productive. She regularly produced about 400 ml of mucoid sputum each day. Breathlessness had become noticeable on relatively mild exertion and she had lost approximately half a stone in weight. The findings on physical examination were essentially unchanged apart from the appearance of scanty late inspiratory crackles in the right middle and lower zones. In

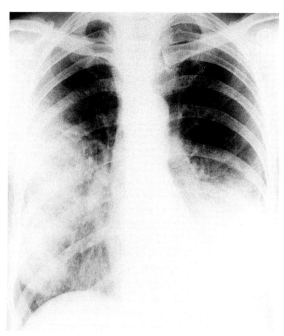

Figure Q10.1

addition to more extensive left-sided consolidation the chest radiograph (Figure Q10.1) now showed widespread patchy shadowing throughout the right lung field.

Questions

1. What is the most likely diagnosis?
2. How might the diagnosis be most readily confirmed?
3. What is the outlook?

Case 11

In the six months leading up to her hospital referral Mrs Isabella MacKie, a 62-year-old housewife, had complained of pain affecting her knees and ankles. Over several visits her general practitioner had failed to note any joint abnormality but had supposed, nevertheless, that her symptoms were due to arthritis and he had prescribed a non-steroidal anti-inflammatory analgesic. A second opinion was arranged when Mrs Mackie presented again with a history of weight loss amounting to about half a stone over the previous three months. She gave no history of any change in her usual 'smoker's cough' and had no complaint of breathlessness. Apart from a history of 'pleurisy' 30 years before she had previously enjoyed robust health. She had smoked 15 cigarettes a day for forty years.

Physical examination revealed gross clubbing affecting the fingers and toes but the hands and feet appeared otherwise normal. However, there were small effusions detectable in both knee joints. There were no abnormal cardiorespiratory findings. The haemoglobin was 11.5 g/dl, white blood cell count 6.5×10^9/l, ESR 31 mm/h. Plasma electrolytes and liver function tests were normal. The serum was positive for rheumatoid factor at a titre of 1/64. The chest X-ray showed a solitary, rounded, soft tissue opacity in the left lower zone. An isotope bone scan showed symmetrically increased uptake affecting the lower femora and the distal parts of the tibiae and fibulae. Fibreoptic bronchoscopy showed no abnormality.

Questions

1. What is the probable clinical diagnosis?
2. What is the significance of the positive bone scan?

Case 12

A 34-year-old bus driver was referred to the chest clinic for investigation of breathlessness. He had first noticed this symptom five years before and had seen his general practitioner on several occasions. The advice was always the same – 'You must stop smoking, Mr Gibson!' Having started to smoke at the age of 12, the habit had grown to the point where he was consuming 60 cigarettes a day. Out of guilt (the general practitioner's advice fell on deaf ears) Mr Gibson's visits to the surgery declined in frequency and, as he had been warned, his breathlessness progressed. By the time he had plucked up enough courage to face his general practitioner again, he found that his effort tolerance was limited to about 200 metres on level ground and that he often had to stop after climbing just a single flight of stairs. Over the previous 18 months Mr Gibson also reported weight loss amounting to about two stones and it was because of this new feature that an outpatient appointment was sought.

When seen in the chest clinic Mr Gibson admitted to daily production of variable quantities of mucopurulent sputum over a period of years. He was sometimes aware of wheeze, especially on exertion, but he denied nocturnal attacks of dyspnoea or wheeze. Despite his history of weight loss he had maintained a normal appetite and he denied any gastrointestinal symptomatology. There was no history of childhood respiratory illness.

At 46 kg Mr Gibson was well below his ideal body weight. There was no evidence of finger clubbing. Breath sounds were strikingly reduced in intensity throughout both lung fields but there were no adventitious sounds. On abdominal examination a smooth liver edge was palpable 6 cm below the costal margin. A chest X-ray showed evidence of hyperinflation and vascular attenuation, particularly in the lower zones. The results of lung function tests are shown in Table Q12.1

Table Q12.1   Results of lung function tests*

	Predicted	Actual	% Predicted
FEV_1	3.80	0.66 (0.68)**	17.4
FVC	4.65	2.74 (2.70)**	58.9
FEV/FVC%	79.1	24.0	30.3
RV	1.80	6.44	357.8
TLC	6.50	10.20	156.9
TL_{co}	10.64	2.87	27.0
K_{co}	1.76	0.40	22.7

* For abbreviations and units, see page x.
** Results after inhaled bronchodilator.

Questions

1. What is the most likely clinical diagnosis?
2. Suggest one confirmatory investigation.
3. What are the implications for Mr Gibson's family?

Case 13

Mrs Marjorie Mayhew, a 52-year-old housewife, was convinced that her 'old TB' had flared up again. Her original pulmonary infection had been diagnosed eight years before, in 1978, when she had felt just as she did now. For 12 months she had been generally unwell, anorexic, intermittently feverish and she had lost about a stone in weight. For some years she had been troubled by a productive cough, but over the previous 12 months this had become more persistent and increasingly productive of purulent or mucopurulent phlegm rather than her usual 'clear spit'. Earlier records showed that her tuberculous infection had been with a fully sensitive strain of *Mycobacterium tuberculosis* and that she had received an adequate duration of therapy which had included rifampicin and isoniazid. Mrs Mayhew was a recent ex-smoker having formerly smoked 15 cigarettes a day since the age of 20.

Physical examination revealed a low grade pyrexia, finger clubbing and extensive signs in the right lung – with patchy impairment of the percussion note, reduction in the intensity of breath sounds and generalized coarse inspiratory crackles.

The haemoglobin was 12.0 g/dl, white blood cell count 13.0×10^9/l, ESR 87 mm/h. The blood urea, creatinine, electrolytes and liver function tests were normal. The plasma globulin was elevated at 42 g/l and protein electrophoresis showed a generalized increase in gammaglobulins. The patient's purulent sputum was repeatedly negative (six specimens) on direct smear for tubercle bacilli but yielded a growth of *Aspergillus fumigatus*. The chest X-ray was reported as follows: 'There are fibrocalcareous changes in both upper zones, more marked on the right side; there is extensive pleural thickening at the right apex where there is also evidence of cavity formation'. Bronchoscopy revealed generalized inflammatory changes throughout the right bronchial tree with moderate amounts of mucopus, but there was no evidence of bronchial obstruction. Sputum (on four occasions) and bronchial aspirate were negative for malignant cells but mycelial elements were identified with ease.

Questions

1. What is the most likely explanation for the patient's clinical deterioration?
2. Suggest two relevant further investigations.

Case 14

Mr Walter Daniel, a 59-year-old security officer, was admitted to the chest unit at his general practitioner's request after a chest film had shown a large pleural effusion. He had presented to the surgery with breathlessness which had first become noticeable four weeks before and which had progressed to the extent that he was dyspnoeic on minimal exertion. He had noted no change in his longstanding cough which was occasionally productive of small amounts of mucoid sputum. He denied any other relevant symptomatology. Mr Daniel was a regular smoker of 20 cigarettes daily. There was no past medical history of note and, in particular, no history of prior respiratory illness. He did however confess to a strong family history of carcinoma of the stomach, both his mother and a sister having died from this cause.

Physical examination was relatively unrewarding, revealing clinical signs consistent with pleural fluid but no other abnormality. In particular he was found to be afebrile with no evidence of lymphadenopathy or hepatosplenomegaly. The chest X-ray showed complete opacification of the right hemithorax with mediastinal displacement to the left; appearances which were interpreted as being due to a massive pleural effusion. Pleural aspiration yielded a white, oily fluid which proved to be a fat-rich exudate (fat content: 36 g/l; protein: 40 g/l). The effusion contained large numbers of lymphocytes and pleural biopsies gave only non-specific findings. No organisms were identified in the pleural fluid and short-term cultures were negative. A tuberculin test was negative at a dilution of 1/1000. The peripheral blood picture was normal.

The pleural effusion rapidly recurred following aspiration but was drained completely following the insertion of an intercostal tube. At this stage repeat PA and lateral view chest radiographs showed clear lung fields but suggested a posterior mediastinal mass which was confirmed on a CT scan. Bronchoscopy and a barium swallow/meal examination showed evidence of tracheal and oesophageal compression/distortion, but there was no intrinsic abnormality affecting the trachea, main airways, oesophagus or stomach.

Questions

1. What is the nature of the pleural fluid ?
2. What is the most likely cause in this patient ?

Case 15

Depending upon the clinical picture, patients with persistent cervical lymphadenopathy may be referred to a variety of hospital clinics for further investigation. Mrs Amanda Terry, a 32-year-old housewife, was seen by a chest physician simply because she was also known to have an abnormal chest X-ray. Nine months before she had noticed two small swellings in the right side of her neck.

Because she had felt well she did not bother to see her general practitioner. She finally went to the surgery only after the original swellings had increased in size. She had also noticed that they were more numerous and that there were now swellings in both sides of her neck.

In his referral letter the general practitioner accurately described Mrs Terry's lymphadenopathy: firm, rubbery, non-tender, discreetly and more or less symmetrically enlarged nodes affecting both deep cervical chains. The nodes had been painless throughout. There was no history of weight loss, sore throat, fever or sweats and Mrs Terry denied any respiratory symptoms. Latterly however she had begun to feel rather more tired than usual. The chest film arranged by the general practitioner is reproduced in Figure Q15.1.

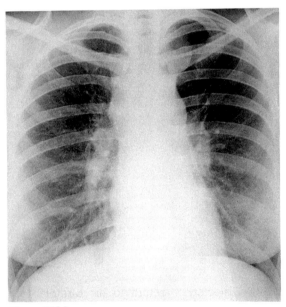

Figure Q15.1

There was no past medical history of note. Mrs Terry was a lifelong non-smoker. She had been given BCG vaccine at the age of thirteen and a healed BCG scar was present. Apart from bilateral cervical lymphadenopathy the only other abnormal physical sign was an enlarged spleen, the tip of which was just palpable. The haemoglobin was 14.6 g/dl, white blood cell count 4.3 × 10^9/l with a normal differential, ESR 47 mm/h. A peripheral blood film showed no abnormality. A tuberculin test (dilution 1/100) gave no induration after 72 hours. The routine plasma biochemical profile was normal except for mild hyperglobulinaemia (38 g/l).

Questions

1. Describe the chest X-ray abnormality.
2. Give the two main differential diagnoses.
3. What is the next diagnostic step?

Case 16 ✓

Having served his joiner's apprenticeship in the Clydeside shipyards in the late 1920s and early 1930s Mr Charles Allen emigrated to the USA in 1936 where he had been gainfully employed as a cabinet-maker. On retiring at the age of 70 he had continued to enjoy excellent health and often boasted that he had never known what it was like to feel ill. Mr Allen was a lifelong non-smoker.

On turning his seventy-fourth birthday, however, he sought medical advice when what he thought had been a simple cold had failed to resolve. Over the previous three months he had suffered a persistent unproductive cough and had become aware of breathlessness on exertion. Despite a normal appetite, he had lost about half a stone in weight. A chest X-ray had apparently suggested a large left pleural effusion and symptomatic improvement followed paracentesis. On being told the results of initial investigations Mr Allen elected to return to his birthplace in Scotland.

An outpatient appointment was secured for Mr Allen shortly after his return to Britain, some six months after the onset of his illness. He now confessed to breathlessness on minimal exertion and persistent, aching left-sided chest pain. On physical examination there was marked dullness to percussion and reduction in breath sounds throughout the left hemithorax. A firm mass measuring about 5 cm in diameter, and fixed to the chest wall, was palpable over the seventh rib interspace in the posterior axillary line. An enlarged lymph node was palpable in the left axilla, but apart from revealing evidence of recent weight loss the remainder of the physical examination was normal.

A chest radiograph showed extensive shadowing in the left lung field with gross circumferential pleural thickening and only a little aerated lung apparent in the left upper zone. The right lung field showed no apparent radiographic abnormality. Pleural aspiration, attempted for therapeutic purposes, revealed a 'dry tap' at each of several sites.

Questions

1. What is the most likely clinical diagnosis?
2. What treatment/s is/are available for this patient?
3. Are there any medicolegal implications?

Case 17

Mrs Margaret Carlyle, a 65-year-old ex-secretary, had been well up to about two months prior to her hospital admission. Over this period she had suffered increasingly severe and more persistent pain in the right shoulder. The pain radiated to the medial aspect of the right upper arm. There was no apparent relation to exertion and the pain was not consistently relieved by simple analgesics or by glyceryl trinitrate, prescribed by her general practitioner. She also admitted to recent weight loss of about one stone and to unaccustomed lethargy. Hospital admission was precipitated by the onset of more severe weakness over the previous 3–4 days, such that she was unable to walk unaided.

There was a long history of chronic cough productive of small amounts of mucoid sputum over many years, but Mrs Carlyle denied being breathless. She was a current smoker of ten cigarettes per day but she had smoked more heavily in the past. There was a five year history of hypertension for which her sole medication was 'Dyazide', one tablet daily. There was also a history of previous pulmonary tuberculosis in the patient's twenties but details of her treatment were not available.

Physical examination revealed evidence of recent weight loss. The blood pressure was 152/94. There was generalized reduction of breath sounds affecting both lung fields but no apparent focal abnormality. Abdominal examination was normal. Neurological examination revealed symmetrically reduced power and diminished sensation affecting all modalities in both lower limbs with absent knee and ankle jerks. There was a right-sided ptosis and miosis.

The haemoglobin was 12.6 g/dl, white blood count 15.2 × 10⁹/l and ESR 130 mm/h. The plasma globulin was elevated at 48 g/l; electroporesis showed a generalized increase in gammaglobulin. A tuberculin test (dilution 1/1000) was negative and sputa were negative on direct smear for tubercle bacilli. The ECG showed non-specific ST/T changes and satisfied voltage criteria for left ventricular hypertrophy. Mrs Carlyle's chest film is reproduced in Figure Q17.1.

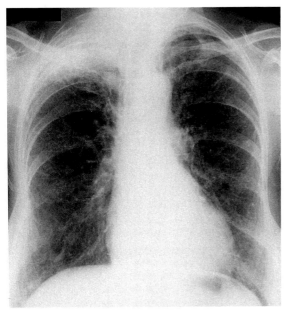

Figure Q17.1

Questions

1. What is the most likely diagnosis?
2. Name three complications that have arisen in this patient.

Case 18 ✓

Mrs Maisy Sands, a 52-year-old housewife, had been perfectly well up until five months before when, following what she had taken to be a simple cold, she developed an irritating unproductive cough. As the months passed her cough persisted and she became increasingly aware of breathlessness on effort. Mrs Sands had attributed this to weight gain (two stones over the previous 18 months) and had not been unduly concerned until she found herself unable to complete her housework without frequent rests. After a visit to the local health centre a chest X-ray was followed by urgent outpatient referral when Mrs Sands' general practitioner had received the X-ray report: 'There is a large area of homogeneous shadowing with a smooth, convex lateral margin in the right paratracheal region. Heart size and silhouette normal. Lung fields clear.'

When seen in the chest clinic Mrs Sands added little of any relevance except that, latterly, she had been aware of 'wheeze' especially on exertion. She said that her appetite was normal. There was no history of febrile symptoms. She denied any previous history of respiratory illness and admitted to having been a lifelong non-smoker.

Mrs Sands was short, stockily built and considerably over-weight. There was no definite cervical abnormality and no obvious superficial lymphadenopathy although the patient's obesity and particularly short neck rendered examination difficult. Noisy inspiratory breath sounds were audible at the mouth but chest auscultation revealed no adventitious sounds.

The haemoglobin was 14.5 g/dl, white blood cell count 6.5×10^9/l, ESR 4 mm/h. A peripheral blood film showed no abnormality. The serum T_3 was 2.0 nmol/l, T_4 97 nmol/l and TSH 0.2 µU/ml. Static and dynamic lung volumes were within normal limits (FEV_1 2.4 l) but the peak expiratory flow rate (200 l/min) was disproportionately low, giving an Empey Index of 12.0.

Questions

1. What is the most likely diagnosis?
2. What is the Empey Index and what is its significance in this case?

Case 19

Jimmy Macgregor was well known in the neighbourhood as the retired local 'bobby'; a 76-year-old bachelor who, according to neighbours, had kept apparently well until about three months before. As the weeks passed Jimmy was seen less and less often around town. He had become less inclined to cook for himself or keep house, but had spurned any offers of help. His neighbours finally called in the general practitioner when, weak and anorexic, he had taken to his bed and refused to move.

After his arrival in the medical ward at the local hospital, Jimmy was unable to give a useful history. He was inattentive, confused, disorientated and gave rambling replies to the houseman's enquiries in a noticeably hoarse voice. According to the general practitioner's referral letter there was no past medical history of note other than longstanding 'chronic bronchitis'.

On physical examination there was clear evidence of marked recent weight loss with nicotine staining of the fingers. Mr Macgregor was clinically dehydrated but afebrile with a heart rate of 84 beats/min in sinus rhythm. The chest was hyperinflated with a generalized reduction in breath sounds, most marked on the left, and expiratory wheeze. There were no focal or lateralizing neurological signs. The optic fundi appeared normal.

The haemoglobin was 10.6 g/dl, white blood cell count 10.8×10^9/l, ESR 106 mm/h. The blood urea was 18.6 mmol, albumin 26 g/l, globulin 48 g/l, calcium (corrected for low albumin) 3.42 mmol/l. Routine urine testing revealed no abnormality. The alkaline phosphatase was 292 IU/l with a normal serum bilirubin and transaminases. A chest X-ray showed low, flat diaphragms but clear lung fields with no bony abnormality; the left hilum appeared abnormally dense. An isotope bone scan was normal.

Questions

1. What is the most likely underlying diagnosis?
2. What treatment should be given?

Case 20

Mrs Annie Morson, an obese 60-year-old widow, was referred to medical outpatients for investigation of breathlessness. In the previous 12 months she had noticed progressive deterioration in effort tolerance to the extent that she was dyspnoeic climbing just one flight of stairs and she had had to reduce her pace on the flat. She slept with two pillows but admitted to waking frequently through the early hours with shortness of breath and wheeze. She also admitted to coughing small amounts of mucoid sputum over the previous year. Mrs Morson had stopped smoking ten years before, having previously smoked about 15 cigarettes a day since the age of 20. Direct questioning elicited a history of angina of effort, of five years duration, as well as longstanding 'heartburn'. Her current medication consisted of atenolol 100 mg daily, cimetidine 800 mg nocte, sublingual glyceryl trinitrate and inhaled salbutamol.

On examination, the cardiac rhythm was regular, rate 84 beats/min, blood pressure 164/90. The apex beat was impalpable and the heart sounds only faintly audible with no obvious added sounds or murmurs. In the chest, there was generalized reduction in the intensity of breath sounds with both inspiratory and expiratory wheeze. The jugular venous pressure was normal.

The haemoglobin was 9.5 g/dl with a hypochromic, microcytic blood picture. Sputum was mucoid and yielded no significant growth. The ECG showed T wave inversion in leads V_5 and V_6 as the only abnormality. A chest X-ray showed significant cardio-megaly with clear lung fields. Skin tests were negative to common inhalant allergens. A barium meal showed a large hiatus hernia and endoscopy revealed severe oesophagitis. The peak flow rate in the clinic was 160 l/min (mean predicted value, 320 l/min), increasing to 210 l/min after inhaled salbutamol. Serial recordings showed an amplitude in PEFR which was about 60% of the average daily reading.

Questions

1. What do you consider to be the most important contributory cause of breathlessness in this patient?
2. What is the implication of this for Mrs Morson's current anti-anginal therapy?

Case 21

Mrs Dorothy Keenan, a 61-year-old housewife, had not felt well for 18 months. She had suffered, what she had taken to be, influenza and ever since had been troubled by a persistent unproductive cough. She decided to seek advice when, over a period of about four months, she had noticed shortness of breath when climbing hills and when carrying heavy shopping. She denied orthopnoea, wheeze, haemoptysis or chest pain but admitted to recent weight loss amounting to about 5 pounds. Mrs Keenan was a regular smoker of 10–15 cigarettes a day. Two years before she had undergone a left mastectomy followed by radiotherapy for carcinoma of the breast but, apart from rheumatic fever at the age of seventeen, there was no other past medical history of note.

On examination she was apyrexial. There was no apparent superficial lymphadenopathy but early finger clubbing was noted. The cardiac rhythm was regular at 68 beats/min and the blood pressure was 140/80. Heart sounds were normal with no added sounds or murmurs. Inspection of the chest revealed a healed mastectomy scar with no evidence of local recurrence and auscultation demonstrated bilateral basal late inspiratory crackles with no other adventitious sounds. Abdominal examination was normal.

The haemoglobin was 14.5 g/dl, WBC 10.3×10^9/l, ESR 6 mm/h. Plasma electrolytes and biochemical tests of liver function were within normal limits. The total protein was elevated at 81 g/l (globulin 39 g/l); plasma protein electrophoresis showed increased α_1 and α_2 globulins as well as a generalized increase in gammaglobulin. The chest X-ray showed bilateral reticulo-nodular shadowing most marked at the lung bases. Lung function tests revealed a mild restrictive ventilatory defect with moderate impairment of total gas transfer. An open lung biopsy subsequently showed a prominent exudate of intra-alveolar macrophages with irregular thickening of alveolar septa and patchy interstitial fibrosis.

Questions

1. What is the likely pathological diagnosis?
2. What treatment is indicated?

Case 22

Mrs Germaine Robertson, a 42-year-old housewife, was admitted to the chest unit after a lower respiratory infection had apparently failed to respond to initial antibiotic therapy. She had been well up until two weeks earlier when she became feverish with a sore throat, headache, earache and general malaise. The symptoms were similar to those her daughter had suffered three weeks before upon her return from boarding school where, it had been reputed, 'there was a bug going around'. Whereas her daughter's illness had resolved within a few days, Mrs Robertson developed a harsh cough productive of only scanty mucopurulent sputum. When seen by her general practitioner, six days after the onset of the illness, she was found to be febrile (38.4°C). The throat appeared infected. There was tender bilateral cervical lymphade-nopathy. The right eardrum was haemorrhagic and inflamed, and coarse inspiratory crackles were audible at the left lung base. She was given a week's course of co-trimoxazole. During the following week Mrs Robertson's upper respiratory symptoms resolved, but her largely unproductive cough persisted and she became aware of breathlessness when carrying out her housework. At this stage the general practitioner secured Mrs Robertson's hospital admission.

Mrs Robertson was an ex-smoker of ten years duration; she had never smoked more than ten cigarettes a day. She had suffered a small left pneumothorax at the age of 24 and a right-sided pneumothorax two years before. On neither occasion was any specific treatment required. Apart from a calf vein thrombosis at the age of eighteen there was no other relevant past medical history.

On admission Mrs Robertson appeared relatively well. She was febrile (38.0°C) and chest auscultation now revealed left basal inspiratory crackles. There was no evidence of finger clubbing, but all of the fingers were noted to be abnormally pale, blue and cold and Mrs Robertson admitted that, for the previous few days, they had been alternately numb and painful. The haemoglobin was 11.9 g/dl, ESR 110 mm/h and white blood count 6.9×10^9/l. The blood film showed a lymphopenia and the presence of large monocytoid cells with deeply staining cytoplasm as well as a mild reticulocytosis. The Paul-Bunnell test was negative. There was a positive Coombs' test and elevated plasma globulins (38 g/l). The patient was unreactive to tuberculin at a dilution of 1/1000 and her

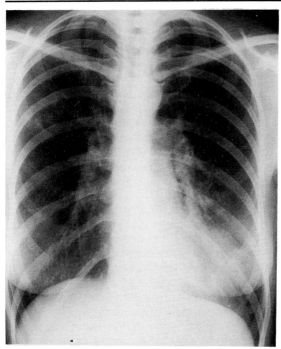

Figure Q22.1

mucopurulent sputum yielded no significant growth. The PA chest X-ray is illustrated in Figure Q22.1.

Questions

1. Describe the radiographic abnormality.
2. What is the most likely diagnosis?
3. Suggest two relevant investigations?

Case 23

Mr Murdo McLeod, a 62-year-old builder, was deemed a good candidate for surgery. He had presented with a four-week history of haemoptysis and a chest X-ray had shown a 4 cm diameter rounded opacity in the left upper lobe. Subesequently, bronchoscopy showed no abnormality but brush biopsies taken under fluoroscopic control showed numerous malignant cells with cytological features in keeping with squamous carcinoma of the bronchus. Despite the fact that he had been a regular smoker lung function tests were within normal limits. Clinical examination and routine biochemistry revealed no evidence of distant metastases. A thoracic CT scan showed no evidence of mediastinal spread and Mr McLeod was therefore referred for a surgical opinion with a view to thoracotomy. Later, at operation, Mr McLeod's tumour was found to transgress the oblique fissure and a left pneumonectomy was carried out.

Postoperatively his early progress was uneventful. Four days after the removal of his chest drain he was apyrexial, mobilizing well but still complaining of a lot of pain from the thoracotomy wound. A chest X-ray showed the expected air-fluid level in the left hemithorax. An ECG was normal. On the tenth postoperative day Mr McLeod was transferred to the chest ward of a hospital nearer his home town for further convalescence. He continued to do well until the day he was due to be discharged when he unexpectedly deteriorated with the sudden onset of severe dyspnoea and cough productive of brownish fluid. He was tachypnoeic and centrally cyanosed with a regular tachycardia of 136 beats/min. The jugular venous pressure was normal. Chest ausculatation revealed coarse crackles throughout the right lung field and signs consistent with a hydropneumothorax on the left. A chest film showed extensive patchy shadowing in the right lung field and, compared with a film two days earlier, the air-fluid level was noted to have fallen.

Questions

1. What complication has occurred?
2. What are the immediate therapeutic requirements?

Case 24

Mr Archibald Ferguson, a 48-year-old garage mechanic, was not happy with his general practitioner's diagnosis of asthma and he insisted on seeing a specialist. He remembered the onset of his illness well. Ten months earlier he had undergone bilateral nasal polypectomy, a procedure which had been carried out on several occasions over the previous ten years. Within a week of the operation he developed a cough with green sputum. There was some improvement following a course of ampicillin but a dry cough persisted and in its wake Mr Ferguson became aware of intermittent breathlessness and wheeze. There had been no history of childhood asthma. Nor was there any family history of asthma, eczema or allergic rhinitis. Mr Ferguson's general practitioner diagnosed late onset 'intrinsic' asthma and he was pleased to note a dramatic response to a short course of oral prednisolone which had apparently rendered the patient essentially asymptomatic. Unfortunately, symptoms recurred within a few weeks of stopping corticosteroids and, despite subsequent treatment with inhaled beclomethasone and salbutamol, Mr Ferguson remained intermittently wheezy and he continued to suffer from an irritating, unproductive cough. Moreover, as the months passed he became generally less well, occasionally feverish and latterly, in the month prior to his clinic referral, he reported weight loss amounting to about half a stone.

When first seen in outpatients Mr Ferguson was found to be mildly febrile (37.6°C) but, otherwise, there were no abnormal physical signs. In particular the chest was clear with no audible adventitious sounds. The haemoglobin was 15.7 g/dl, white blood count 10.9×10^9/l with the following differential: 56% neutrophils, 16% lymphocytes, 3% monocytes and 24% eosinophils. The ESR was 110 mm/h. A wide range of skin tests to common inhalant allergens, including *Aspergillus fumigatus*, was negative and the total serum IgE level was normal. A battery of serological tests revealed no evidence of parasitic infestation. Pulmonary function tests (static and dynamic lung volumes, single breath gas transfer) were within normal limits but the chest film revealed a striking abnormality: extensive, symmetrical, homogeneous areas of shadowing occupying the peripheral parts of both lung fields.

Questions

1. What is the clinical diagnosis?
2. What treatment is necessary?

Case 25

Mrs Lillian Sales, a 46-year-old former nurse, was referred to respiratory outpatients by her general practitioner with a relatively short history of paroxysmal attacks of breathlessness and wheeze which had been unresponsive to a variety of bronchodilator treatments. She was seen by the senior house officer who obtained a history, over the previous four weeks, of increasing symptomatology culminating in urgent outpatient referral. The referral letter indicated that despite her severe symptoms and, latterly, her inability to carry out housework Mrs Sales had always managed to attend the surgery and there had been no requests for house calls.

Mrs Sales appeared distressed but was able to carry out a conversation easily. The resting cardiac rate was 96 beats/min. Inspiratory and expiratory wheeze was readily audible with the unaided ear but the senior house officer was puzzled when, using the stethoscope applied to the chest wall, wheezing sounded 'distant'. Without more ado, in a busy outpatient clinic, Mrs Sales was admitted to the ward and the houseman was instructed to administer nebulized salbutamol (5 mg), intravenous hydrocortisone (200 mg), 35% oxygen and to organize a chest X-ray and arterial blood gases.

Later in the afternoon the SHO visited the patient with the senior registrar when the houseman related Mrs Sales' extensive past medical history. Five years before she had undergone a right nephrectomy for pyelonephritis. Two years later a hysterectomy had been carried out for menorrhagia. There was a previous history of depressive illness. There was no history of childhood asthma. Twelve months prior to her hospital admission she had suffered a mild right hemiplegia (there was a strong family history of cerebrovascular disease) but had subsequently made a full functional recovery. Mrs Sales had retired on the grounds of ill health at the time of her stroke. She was a regular smoker of 20 cigarettes per day.

Despite her initial therapy Mrs Sales appeared much as she had done in the clinic. A PA chest film showed no abnormality and the blood gases showed that she was normocapnic (P_{CO_2} 5.20 kPa). Subsequently, inspiratory and expiratory flow volume curves, while the patient was still symptomatic, showed changes consistent with a variable extrathoracic obstruction. Symptoms were relieved by inhalation of a gas mixture consisting of 80% helium and 20% oxygen. Fibreoptic bronchoscopy was carried out

48 hours after admission, when Mrs Sales was asymptomatic. No abnormality was demonstrated in either the upper or the lower respiratory tract.

Questions

1. What is the most likely explanation for Mrs Sales' respiratory symptoms?
2. How might bronchoscopic examination have contributed to this diagnosis?

Case 26

Mr Reginald MacCutcheon, a 57-year-old crofter, had been well until about six months before when he had presented to his general practitioner with a short history of breathlessness on exertion. He was found to be both overweight and significantly hypertensive (180/110) whereupon treatment was instituted with a calcium antagonist. Over the next six months Mr MacCutcheon became progressively more dyspnoeic. Medical referral followed when, after the addition of a regular diuretic to his antihypertensive therapy, there had been no clear clinical improvement.

When first seen in the clinic Mr MacCutcheon admitted to an effort tolerance of about 150 metres on the flat. In the previous six months he had noted intermittent 'hoarseness' and he had become increasingly aware of marked shortness of breath whenever he lay flat, although there there was no history of specifically nocturnal attacks of dyspnoea. He denied chest pain, ankle swelling, cough or haemoptysis. He was a lifelong non-smoker. Apart from his recently diagnosed hypertension there was no past history of note.

Mr MacCutcheon was moderately obese and spoke in a weak voice. Although he was not apparently breathless sitting at rest, he became distressed on adopting the recumbent position. The cardiac rhythm was regular, rate 90 beats/min, blood pressure 170/100. The heart sounds were normal with no added sounds or murmurs. In the chest, breath sounds were reduced especially at the lung bases but there were no adventitious sounds. The jugular venous pressure was normal and there was no dependent oedema. Neurological examination revealed coarse fasiculation in all limbs up to the level of C_5 and weakness of lower motor neurone type with some wasting of the small muscles of the left hand. Ankle jerks were absent but other limb reflexes were brisk and symmetrical. The plantar responses were flexor and there were no abnormal sensory signs.

The haemoglobin was 16.9 g/dl, white blood count 11.4×10^9/l, ESR 2 mm/h. The serum creatine phosphokinase was normal. A chest X-ray showed a normal cardiac size and silhouette. Both hemidiaphragms were elevated and there were bi-basal shadows of 'linear atelectasis'. An ECG showed no abnormality. Pulmonary function tests showed a mild restrictive ventilatory defect. The flow-volume curve demonstrated reduced flows at all lung volumes with a particularly flat inspiratory limb. The FVC which was 2.2 litres in the erect position (predicted value 3.9 litres) fell to 0.4 litres when the test was repeated with Mr MacCutcheon lying supine. The K_{co} was 140% of the predicted value.

Questions

1. What is the probable clinical diagnosis?
2. What is the explanation for Mr MacCutcheon's marked orthopnoea?
3. How might this be verifed?

Case 27

Mrs Jane Hammond, a 66-year-old non-smoker, had enjoyed poor health for some time. She had suffered from angina for three years. Eighteen months before she had been an inpatient following a confirmed inferior myocardial infarct. Her hospital stay was complicated by pulmonary embolism. She had also been hypertensive for ten years, but it had been found possible to withdraw all antihypertensive therapy after her infarct and for some months her only medication had consisted of diuretics (frusemide 40 mg and amiloride 5 mg daily).

This time it was the surgical ward to which she was admitted with a 24-hour history of lower abdominal pain and vomiting. There had been a background of intermittent rectal bleeding over the previous two months. The findings on physical examination and the results of abdominal films were in keeping with large bowel obstruction. This diagnosis was confirmed at laparotomy which revealed a large tumour of the descending colon. A left hemicolectomy and defunctioning transverse colostomy were carried out.

Mrs Hammond's initial postoperative progress was uneventful. On the second postoperative day, however, she became pyrexial (39.2°C), hypotensive (70/40) and oliguric (urine output 10 ml/h). A chest X-ray at this stage showed mild cardiomegaly with clear lung fields. The ECG showed evidence of previous inferior infarction and a sinus tachycardia as the only abnormalities. The total white blood cell count was $22.0 \times 10^9/l$ and blood cultures subsequently yielded a growth of gram-negative bacilli. Clinical improvement followed treatment with intravenous fluids and broad spectrum antibiotic therapy but a low-dose dopamine infusion was required to maintain a urine output > 40 ml/h.

On the third postoperative day Mrs Hammond was apyrexial but her condition deteriorated once again. She became increasingly dyspnoeic over the course of the next 24 hours. She denied chest pain and was producing only small quantities of mucoid sputum. She was tachypneoic with a tachycardia of 130 beats/min, blood pressure 120/74. There were bi-basal late inspiratory lung crackles. ECG appearances were unchanged from those two days before. The chest X-ray showed bilateral alveolar infiltrates. Arterial blood gases (F_{IO_2} 0.6–60%) yielded a Pa_{O_2} of 5.86 kPa and a Pa_{CO_2} of 3.73 kPa with a moderate metabolic acidoisis. A Swan-Ganz catheter gave a pulmonary capillary wedge pressure of 1.33 kPa (10 mmHg).

Questions

1. What is the reason for Mrs Hammond's deterioration?
2. What is the prognosis?
3. How should respiratory failure be managed in this patient?

Case 28

Jimmy Provan, a 29-year-old bank clerk, was a regular attender at the rheumatology clinic. His joint problem had started about two years earlier with pain and stiffness principally affecting the elbows, wrists and metacarpo-phalangeal joints of both hands and, to a lesser extent, both knees and ankles. On the whole his symptoms had been well controlled with naproxen and, latterly, he had tended to miss his clinic appointments. In the previous two months, however, he had been less well and had phoned the clinic asking whether he might be seen earlier than had been arranged.

When seen later that week he gave a two-month history of breathlessness noticeable on moderate exertion. For a similar period he had felt generally unwell and intermittently feverish with some loss of appetite and weight loss amounting to about six pounds. His joint symptoms had been a little more troublesome than usual but he had been able to continue at work without any difficulty. In the previous four weeks he had developed a cough productive of scanty mucoid sputum. There was no history of chest pain or haemoptysis. Jimmy was a regular smoker of about 15 cigarettes a day.

On examination, he was pyrexial (38.2°C) and appeared pale and unwell. There was some synovial swelling and tenderness affecting the wrists and metacarpo-phalangeal joints of both hands, and small effusions were present in both knee joints. There were no subcutaneous nodules. In the chest there was dullness to percussion and marked reduction in breath sounds in the right middle and lower zones. There were no adventitious sounds.

The haemoglobin was 11.0 g/dl with a normocytic blood picture, white blood count 9.9×10^9/l, ESR 62 mm/h. Routine biochemical tests were normal except for raised plasma globulins (45 g/l). Sputum specimens were unobtainable. Serum was positive for rheumatoid factor at a titre of 1/320. The chest X-ray showed a moderate right pleural effusion with patchy shadowing and irregular cavitation at the right apex. A diagnostic pleural tap revealed slightly turbid, straw-coloured fluid with a protein content of 43 g/l and sugar content of 1.6 mmol/l. Cytological examination showed numerous lymphocytes and no malignant cells. Short term cultures of the pleural fluid were sterile.

Questions

1. What is the most likely explanation for the pleural effusion?
2. What other investigations are indicated?

Case 29

Mr Pottinger, a 60-year-old company director, was referred for further assessment after an insurance examination had disclosed abnormal biochemical tests of liver function. He himself complained only of lethargy over the previous three months and he denied any respiratory symptoms. He was an ex-smoker of three years' duration, having previously smoked 20 cigarettes a day, but he admitted to a heavy alcohol intake. On examination, there were cutaneous stigmata of chronic liver disease with moderate splenomegaly. There were no abnormal respiratory findings and no evidence of superficial lymphadenopathy, but the chest film showed marked widening of the mediastinum. The lung fields were clear.

A liver biopsy showed established cirrhotic changes and other features favouring an alcoholic aetiology. Mediastinoscopy and biopsy of the enlarged lymph nodes showed infiltration by 'lymphocyte depleted' Hodgkin's disease. Bone marrow examination was normal but lymphangiography and abdominal CT showed extensive involvement of lymph nodes in both iliac and para-aortic chains (clinical stage III A). The treatment plan was to consist of alternating courses of MOPP (mustine, vincristine, procarbazine, prednisolone) and ABVD (adriamycin, bleomycin, vinblastine, DTIC). Pretreatment blood counts were within normal limits.

The first course of MOPP was tolerated well with nadir white blood cell and platelet counts of $3.1 \times 10^9/l$ and $54 \times 10^9/l$ respectively, but with lymphopenia noted in the blood film. Peripheral counts had recovered before the first course of ABVD to which Mr Pottinger reacted with fever and rigors. When he was reviewed in outpatients two weeks later he appeared well, but said he had become aware of progressive breathlessness since his last course of treatment to the extent that he was dyspnoeic on mild exertion. He had also developed an unproductive cough.

On examination, he was tachypnoeic at rest but not cyanosed (Pa_{O_2} 9.60 kPa, Pa_{CO_2} 1.87 kPa). There was a low grade pyrexia. The chest was clear on auscultation but the chest film showed bilateral, diffuse 'alveolar' consolidation. The mediastinum now appeared normal. The heart size was within normal limits and the ECG showed no abnormality. An abdominal film showed a marked reduction in size of the nodes noted to have been enlarged in the earlier lymphangiogram. The spleen remained markedly enlarged. The haemoglobin was 11.6 g/dl, white blood count

$6.7 \times 10^9/l$ (normal differential), platelets $322 \times 10^9/l$. Pulmonary function tests showed moderate restriction with about 2.8 litres loss of lung capacity with a reduced K_{co}. Induced sputum and blood cultures were sterile.

Questions

1. What is the differential diagnosis of the pulmonary infiltration?
2. Which of the cytotoxic drugs might be implicated?

Case 30

Mrs Agnes Reeves, a 64-year-old housewife and a heavy cigarette smoker, gave a ten-year history of ulcerative colitis. She had been maintained on treatment with sulphasalazine and, apart from minor exacerbations which had never required hospital admission, she had generally remained well. Her general practitioner became concerned, however, when following an influenza-like illness Mrs Reeves did not pick up. Over a period of two to three weeks she reported weight loss of about one stone associated with an increase in stool frequency and, in the 24 hours prior to admission, frank bloody diarrhoea. Despite intensive medical therapy, Mrs Reeves remained acutely unwell with blood-stained diarrhoea 10–12 times per day and persistent pyrexia. Forty-eight hours after admisssion her condition deteriorated markedly with increased abdominal pain and the erect abdominal film showed free intra-abdominal gas. Subsequent laparotomy confirmed total colitis and a small perforation was demonstrated at the splenic flexure. A total colectomy was carried out and an ileostomy was fashioned.

Mrs Reeves had a stormy postoperative course. She was markedly hypoalbuminaemic (22 g/l) and parenteral nutrition was instituted. She continued to suffer a low grade fever, her abdominal wound became infected and on the seventh postoperative day she developed signs of a left deep venous thrombosis (DVT). A wound swab grew *Staphylococcus aureus,* blood cultures were sterile and venography confirmed the clinical diagnosis of DVT. Heparin was given by intravenous infusion (substituted with warfarin after five days) and adequate wound drainage was secured. By the fourteenth postoperative day there had been clear improvement. The wound was clean, her temperature had settled, her appetite had returned and parenteral feeding was discontinued.

A medical opinion was requested when, two days later, she deteriorated once again with the onset of left-sided pleuritic chest pain. She was pyrexial (38°C) with a tachycardia of 110 beats/min. Her sputum container revealed heavily bloodstained yellow sputum. There was an area dullness to percussion anteriorly in the left mid-zone with bronchial breath sounds. The right lung field was clear. The ECG showed a sinus tachycardia as the only abnormality. The haemoglobin was 12.9 g/dl, white blood count 23 × 10⁹/l, platelets, 701 × 10⁹/l, ESR 88 mm/h. The prothrombin time was 36 s (control 12 s). The chest film is shown in Figure Q30.1. A preoperative chest film had shown no abnormality.

Questions

1. Describe the radiographic abnormality.
2. What is the most likely cause of Mrs Reeves' deterioration?

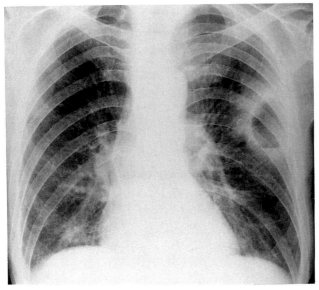

Figure Q30.1

Case 31

Mr Frank Jamieson, a 38-year-old labourer, was admitted to a general surgical ward in the early hours of New Year's Day. He had been drinking heavily and was unable to give a coherent history. According to his friend he had seemed well earlier in the evening but he had undoubtedly had too much to drink. The friend recalled that, towards the end of the evening, he had found Mr Jamieson in the toilet where he had been vomiting. He appeared pale, was perspiring freely and complained of severe pain in the upper abdomen and back. Immediate hospital transfer was arranged.

Mr Jamieson was well known for his history of alcohol abuse, having been admitted to the medical ward on several occasions over the previous five years for symptoms related to alcohol withdrawal. He had been investigated for dyspepsia six months before when upper gastrointestinal endoscopy had shown marked oesophago-gastritis. He had since taken cimetidine on an intermittent basis. He was a regular smoker of 30 cigarettes a day.

On arrival in the ward Mr Jamieson was disorientated and confused. He was distressed, tachypnoeic and obviously in pain. He had a tachycardia of 120 beats/min and a blood pressure of 150/100. The chest was clear on auscultation but there was tenderness over the left lower chest posteriorly. In the abdomen there was some epigastric tenderness but no guarding and bowel sounds were present. The ECG showed a sinus tachycardia but no specific abnormality. Erect and supine abdominal films were normal. The chest X-ray showed a small, left basal, pleural effusion. The haemoglobin was 16.4 g/dl, white blood count 19.8 $\times$ 10^9/l, blood urea 5.3 mmol/l, creatinine 98 μmol/l, sodium 138 mmol/l, potassium 3.5 mmol/l, amylase 160 IU/l, alcohol 267 mg/100 ml.

Mr Jamieson was given analgesia and observed overnight. By the following morning he had become pyrexial (38.0°C). He showed a persistent sinus tachycardia (130 beats/min) and had now developed signs at the left lung base with dullness to percussion and diminished breath sounds. A repeat chest X-ray showed a left hydropneumothorax and a medical opinion was requested.

Questions

1. What is the clinical diagnosis?
2. How should this be confirmed?

Case 32

Mr Allan Williamson, a 45-year-old shopkeeper, had been referred to rheumatology outpatients primarily for the assessment of his complaint – over the previous two months – of pain and stiffness affecting both knees, the elbows and the right wrist. However, he readily confessed to a variety of extra-articular symptoms. He had noted that he tired much more readily than usual and, for about six weeks, he had suffered an irritating unproductive cough and unaccustomed breathlessness on exertion. Over the same period he had lost half a stone in weight. He denied haemoptysis or wheeze and gave no history of previous respiratory illness.

Mr Williamson was an ex-smoker of seven years' duration, but he had smoked 15 cigarettes a day prior to this. He admitted to a period of heavy alcohol abuse after his wife's death four years before but said that he had been totally abstinent in the previous 12 months. Apart from surgery for varicose veins many years before there was no past medical history of note.

On examination he was pyrexial (38.2°C). He appeared anaemic and unwell. He was dyspnoeic with the effort of undressing. The cardiac rhythm was regular, rate 92 beats/min, arterial pressure 162/100. There were no cardiac murmurs. A few coarse inspiratory crackles were noted at the left lung base. Small effusions were detectable in both knee joints, but no other joint abnormality was demonstrable. There were a few scattered purpuric skin lesions (0.5 cm diameter) distributed around the ankles and over some of his fingers. The venous pressure was normal and there was no dependent oedema. Abdominal examination revealed no abnormality.

Urinalysis revealed 3+ protein and 2+ blood. The haemoglobin was 7.4 g/dl, white blood count $17.6 \times 10^9/l$ (78% neutrophils, 10% lymphocytes, 7% monocytes, 5% eosinophils, 1% basophils), platelets $792 \times 10^9/l$, ESR 140 mm/h. A midstream urine specimen showed red cells and both hyaline and granular cats in the spun deposit. The routine biochemistry was normal except for the blood urea (8.7 mmol/l) and creatinine (277 μmol/l); five days later the values were 14.2 mmol/l and 344 μmol/l, respectively. The 24 hour urine volume was 1.6 litres and the creatinine clearance 29 ml/min. Tests for serum rheumatoid factor and antinuclear factor were negative. Venous blood cultures (4 sets) were sterile.

The chest X-ray is shown in Figure Q32.1. Lung function tests showed a moderate restrictive ventilatory defect with about 2.4 litres loss of lung capacity. The K_{co} (corrected for blood haemoglobin concentration) was 124% of the predicted normal value. Arterial blood gases revealed moderate arterial hypoxaemia (Pao_2 6.53 kPa with a $Paco_2$ of 3.46 kPa and pH of 7.52).

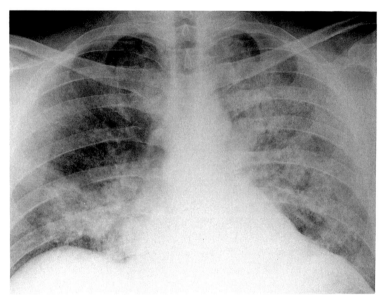

Figure Q32.1

Questions

1. Mr Williamson's illness may not appear to conform to any particular syndrome, but what pathological process best accounts for the clinical picture?
2. How would you confirm the diagnosis?
3. What treatment is required?

Case 33

A 58-year-old patient, Mrs Jean Harrison – a 'lollipop lady' at the local school – gave a long history of bronchial asthma dating from early childhood. She had suffered repeated hospitalization and considerable loss of schooling up to the age of about sixteen, but her symptoms had been less severe during early adult life. In the previous four years, however, she had noticed a recurrence of more troublesome symptoms especially during the winter months. She was a lifelong non-smoker. Her regular medication consisted of inhaled beclomethasone and salbutamol.

For the first time in many years she now found herself back in hospital when, true to form, she had developed increased breathlessness and wheeze during a particularly cold spell of winter weather. She normally produced small quantities of mucoid sputum, but in the week prior to admission her sputum had become purulent. She was pyrexial and tachypnoeic with a tachyardia of 120 beats/min and an unrecordable peak flow rate. A harsh systolic ejection murmur was heard loudest at the left sternal edge with transmission to the neck, arterial pressure 188/92. The haemoglobin was 13.8 g/dl and the white blood count 7.6 × 10⁹/l with a normal differential. Sputum yielded a growth of *Haemophilus influenzae*. The chest X-ray (Figure Q33.1) showed fibrotic changes in both upper lobes and calcified left hilar lymph nodes, although there was no definite history of previous tuberculosis.

Progressive improvement followed treatment with nebulized bronchodilator therapy, systemic steroids and a broad spectrum antibiotic. The peak flow rate climbed to around 320 l/min after five days when Mrs Harrison was allowed home to complete a course of prednisolone over the next fortnight. When seen in the clinic a month later she was 'back to her usual self' and had started back to work.

Two months later, however, hospital admission was requested once again. She had been well up to about four weeks before apart from one mild exacerbation of asthma managed by her general practitioner with a short course of prednisolone. Latterly, however, she had become anorexic with weight loss of one stone. Her husband had noticed a change in her personality and she had become lethargic, apathetic and intermittently confused. On admission she was found to be pyrexial (38.4°C) and disorientated. There were no focal chest signs, nor any focal or lateralizing neurological signs. A loud systolic ejection murmur was again

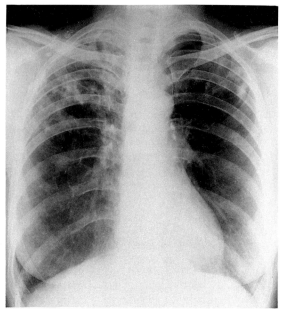

Figure Q33.1

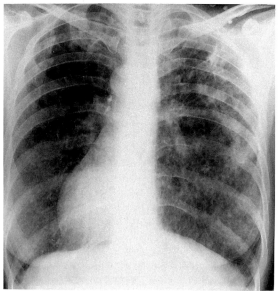

Figure Q33.2

audible. The haemoglobin was 10.8 g/dl, white blood count 5.0 × 10⁹/l, ESR 94 mm/h. The routine biochemical profile was normal apart from raised plasma globulins (42 g/l). Lumbar puncture yielded normal CSF. Initial blood cultures (3 sets) were sterile. The chest film at this stage is shown in Figure Q33.2.

Questions

1. What change has occurred in the most recent chest X-ray?
2. What is the probable clinical diagnosis?

Case 34

Mr Henry Masters, a 52-year-old bachelor, was referred for a medical opinion after he had seen a solicitor about his firm belief, inflamed by recent publicity, that he had asbestos-related disease. For about eight years Mr Masters had been aware of shortness of breath. This had progressed to the extent that he claimed the need to stop after climbing two flights of stairs and that his effort tolerance was limited to about a quarter of a mile on the level. He had felt that his breathlessness was the reason for his other main complaint, that of feeling persistently tired and especially sleepy at work and when driving. He had fallen asleep at the wheel on one occasion. He returned from work feeling 'exhausted' and regularly fell asleep in front of the television: he said he had 'never seen the end of a film yet'. He admitted to a regular cough productive of mucoid and, occasionally, mucopurulent sputum on most days for many years. He denied orthopnoea or nocturnal attacks of dyspnoea but complained that he slept poorly, waking about six times each night to pass urine. His wife's complaint was that he snored loudly and they had had to sleep apart for this reason.

Mr Masters worked as a painter and recalled a period of absestos exposure lasting eighteen months, ten years before, when he had been engaged on painting several large blocks of flats. He had never handled asbestos himself but he had worked in the vicinity of men using finished asbestos products throughout the buildings. He was a regular smoker of 20 cigarettes a day and drank about about a quarter of a bottle of whisky a day. He had been diagnosed as hypertensive six years before. His only medication consisted of bendrofluazide, 5 mg daily.

On examination Mr Masters was obese. There was no evidence of finger clubbing. The cardiac rhythm was regular, 88 beats/min and the blood pressure 168/96. In the chest breath sounds were generally diminished with expiratory polyphonic wheeze and some coarse, early inspiratory bi-basal crackles. A chest X-ray showed no abnormality. Lung function tests showed moderate impairment of dynamic lung volumes with slight improvement following inhaled bronchodilator. The lungs were hyperinflated, the TLC being 130% of the predicted normal value. Total gas transfer was within normal limits.

Questions

1. Is there any evidence of absbestos-related disease?
2. What respiratory problems does Mr Masters have?
3. What further investigations are indicated?

Case 35

Radiographic evidence of lobar collapse in an elderly smoker frequently carries a sinister implication and always merits early investigation. Mrs Winifred Eastcliffe, a 65-year-old widow, was therefore referred for urgent outpatient assessment on the basis of the following X-ray report: 'There is collapse-consolidation of the right upper lobe with increased density of the right hilum, consistent with bronchial neoplasm.' The chest film had been arranged by her general practitioner after an apparent lower respiratory infection had failed to resolve. One month earlier she had developed febrile symptoms with pleuritic right-sided chest pain and cough which, despite treatment with separate courses of amoxycillin and erythromycin, remained productive of small amounts of tenacious yellow sputum.

There was a longstanding history of breathlessness and wheeze dating back to Mrs Eastcliffe's childhood. However, in latter years, these symptoms had been less evident and although she had been prescribed beclomethasone and salbutamol inhalers she confessed that she rarely used them. She had suffered a productive cough for several years but usually only during the winter months. There was no history of haemoptysis.

Mrs Eastcliffe admitted to six previous episodes of 'pneumonia' over the previous ten years and she had been followed at a chest clinic in another part of the country for much of this time. Being relatively new to the area, however, her previous records were not available. Apart from longstanding perennial rhinitis and chronic, predominantly flexural eczema there was no other past medical history of note. Mrs Eastcliffe was a regular smoker, but she had never smoked more than five cigarettes a day. There was a strong family history of asthma.

When seen in outpatients she was apyrexial. There was no evidence of finger clubbing . Physical signs in the chest were consistent with the reported radiographic abnormality; there was no audible wheeze. The peak flow rate was 320 l/min. A repeat chest X-ray two weeks after the initial film continued to show right upper lobe collapse-consolidation, but additional left-sided perihilar consolidation was also evident. The haemoglobin was 15.0 g/dl, white blood count 10.4×10^9/l with the following differential: neutrophils 56%, lymphocytes 20%, monocytes 7%, eosinophils 13%.

Questions

1. What is the most likely underlying diagnosis?
2. Suggest two therapeutic measures relevant to this patient.

Case 36

Mrs Jean Graham, a 61-year-old housewife, was admitted to the medical unit at her general practitioner's request. She had been well until about two months prior to admission. During this period she had been aware of a persistent unproductive cough and increasing shortness of breath. The latter symptom had progressed to the extent that breathlessness was apparent on mild physical exertion. She denied nocturnal dyspnoea or wheeze and gave no history of chest pain or ankle swelling. Latterly Mrs

Graham's husband had become increasingly concerned about his wife's extreme lethargy. He had also noted that she was abnormally drowsy and intermittently confused.

There was a previous history of cholecystectomy eight years earlier and hypertension of six years' duration. Mrs Graham had stopped smoking two years before, having smoked 30 cigarettes a day prior to this. Her medication consisted of methyldopa (250 mg tid) and 'Moduretic' (one tablet daily).

On examination she was apyrexial. The cardiac rhythm was regular, rate 86 beats/min, arterial pressure 174/90. The apex beat was displaced in the anterior axillary line. The aortic second sound was loud but there were no added sounds or murmurs. The lung fields were clear on auscultation. A firm, slightly tender liver edge was palpable 10 cm below the right costal margin. The optic fundi showed some narrowing and increased tortuosity of arterioles but no other abnormality.

Routine laboratory results were as follows: haemoglobin 15.1 g/dl, white blood count $11.2 \times 10^9/l$, platelets $86 \times 10^9/l$, ESR 10 mm/h. The blood film showed a leuco-erythroblastic picture. The blood urea was 2.4 mmol/l, creatinine 50 μmol/l, sodium 110 mmol/l, potassium 3.1 mmol/l, chloride 86 moml/l, AST 126 IU/l, ALT 154 IU/l, alkaline phosphatase 356 IU/l. The chest X-ray showed cardiomegaly, widening of the right superior mediastinum and loss of definition of the right heart border. An isotope brain scan showed no abnormality.

Questions

1. What is the probable diagnosis?
2. How would you confirm this and where would you expect to find the primary abnormality?
3. What is the most likely explanation for
   (a) the electrolyte abnormalities and
   (b) the haematological abnormalities?

Case 37

Jeremy Sissons, an unemployed 18-year-old, gave a long history of respiratory problems. He had been told by his parents that he had been a 'chesty child' and he had suffered several episodes of 'pleurisy' and 'pneumonia' during his primary school years. For a period in his early 'teens his chest symptoms had been somewhat less troublesome. In the previous three years, however, his cough had become more persistent and increasingly productive with about half a cupful of yellow sputum daily. Over the same period he had noted intermittent haemoptysis and for twelve months he had been aware of breathlessness climbing stairs. Despite a normal appetite he had lost nearly a stone in weight over the previous 1–2 years. He denied any recent change in bowel habit but volunteered that for some years he had tended to pass rather pale stools. Apart from an appendicectomy at the age of 14 there was no other past medical history of note. Being an adopted child, Jeremy was unaware of his family history. He had regularly smoked ten cigarettes a day for three years.

On examination, Jeremy appeared pale and thin. The fingers were clubbed. The chest appeared hyperinflated. The percussion note was generally hyper-resonant and auscultation revealed bilateral upper and mid-zone crackles with a few scattered monophonic wheezes. Abdominal examination was normal. The haemoglobin was 11.6 g/dl, white blood count 8.8 × 10^9/l, ESR 34 mm/h. The serum albumin was 31 g/l . Immunoglobulin levels were normal except for a moderately elevated IgG. The sputum yielded a heavy growth of 'mucoid' *Pseudomonas aeruginosa*. Skin tests to common inhalant allergens gave negative results. Avian and aspergillus precipitins were also negative. The chest X-ray confirmed the presence of hyperinflation and showed parallel-line shadows in both upper zones. Pulmonary function tests showed a moderately severe obstructive ventilatory defect.

Questions

1. What is the most likely clinical diagnosis?
2. Suggest two relevant investigations.

Case 38

Despite treatment with a variety of analgesics Mrs Cox, a 54-year-old barmaid, was troubled by persistent chest pain. At the outset, three months before, the pain had been intermittent but for several weeks she had suffered more or less continuous left submammary aching pain which was worse when she coughed and when lying flat. She had occasionally been aware of discomfort in the left shoulder and left upper arm. Her general practitioner requested a respiratory opinion after a chest X-ray arranged at the local casualty department was reported as showing marked elevation of the left hemidiaphragm with loss of definition of the left heart border.

When seen in the chest clinic Mrs Cox admitted to recent lethargy and malaise with weight loss of about one stone. She also confessed to a longstanding smoker's cough although, for some weeks, this had been more persistent than usual. For two months she had also been aware of breathlessness when climbing hills or when carrying heavy shopping. She was a regular smoker of 40 cigarettes a day. She had had medical treatment for a duodenal ulcer five years before, but she denied any recent history of dyspepsia. Apart from treatment for an 'anxiety state' following her divorce three years earlier there was no past history of note.

On examination, Mrs Cox looked unwell and showed evidence of obvious recent weight loss. The cardiac rhythm was regular, rate 82 beats/min, blood pressure 154/80. Chest expansion was diminished on the left with dullness to percussion and reduced breath sounds at the left base. The haemoglobin was 13.0 g/dl, white blood count 10.4×10^9/l, ESR 37 mm/h. An ECG showed no abnormality. Screening of the left hemidiaphragm showed paradoxical movement. Fibreoptic bronchoscopy was normal. A repeat chest film was reported as showing no change.

While awaiting diagnostic thoracotomy Mrs Cox deteriorated rapidly. Her general practitioner requested hospital admission when, over a period of three to four days, she became increasingly breathless. When seen in the ward she was dyspnoeic at rest with a sinus tachycardia of 120 beats/min, a low volume pulse and a blood pressure of 90/60. The physical findings in the chest were essentially unchanged except that the heart sounds were faint and the jugular venous pressure markedly elevated. The chest film showed an increase in the size of the cardiac silhouette compared with earlier films, but the lung fields were unchanged. The ECG showed low voltage complexes with generalized non-specific T wave changes.

Questions

1. What is the probable underlying diagnosis?
2. What complication accounts for Mrs Cox's rapid clinical deterioration?

Case 39

Bill Jessop, a 56-year-old farm worker, had always considered that he had led a healthy life, having been born and brought up in the country and never having smoked so much as a single cigarette. He had also prided himself on his physical fitness and it came as an unpleasant surprise when, over the previous 18 months, he had found himself increasingly breathless on exertion. At first, shortness of breath had been intermittent but, for three months, breathlessness had been more persistent. His effort tolerance had greatly diminished and he had found increasing difficulty in coping with work on the farm. For a short period a salbutamol inhaler, prescribed by his general practitioner, had given some relief but despite its regular use shortness of breath increased in severity. He returned to the surgery for further advice after a series of evenings at home when he had been dyspnoeic at rest. Mr Jessop was advised to remain off work and a chest clinic appointment was secured for later that week.

On going over the history in the clinic Mr Jessop admitted that his breathlessness had tended to be most troublesome in the evenings. He had also been aware of breathlessness during the day, especially after work in the barn where he had often noted sneezing and lachrymation. He lived on the farm and had noticed no change in his symptoms at weekends, but he had suffered no trouble at all six months before when he and his wife had spent a fortnight's holiday in Blackpool. He denied any febrile symptoms or weight loss but admitted to a dry cough, especially at night, in the previous three months.

Table Q37.1 Results of lung function tests*

	Predicted	Actual	% predicted
FEV_1	2.87	1.40 (1.54)**	48.8
FVC	3.88	2.12 (2.34)**	54.1
FEV/FVC%	70	66	94.3
RV	2.07	4.10	198.1
TLC	5.80	6.26	107.9
RV/TLC%	35.7	68.0	190.5
TL_{co}	8.54	8.35	97.8
K_{co}	1.44	1.92	133.3

* For abbreviations and units, see page x.
** Results after inhaled bronchodilator.

Mr Jessop was breathless with the effort of undressing. He was apyrexial with no evidence of finger clubbing. The pulse was regular, rate 90 beats/min, blood pressure 135/80. In the chest breath sounds were generally diminished in intensity. There were no adventitious sounds other than a few scattered monophonic expiratory wheezes. A chest X-ray showed no abnormality. Lung function results are shown in Table Q37.1.

Questions

1. What is the clinical diagnosis?
2. What clinical investigation might you employ to confirm this diagnosis.

Case 40

A 17-year-old schoolgirl was seen at the local Accident and Emergency Department after slipping on an icy path. She had fallen on her left side and complained of pain around the shoulder

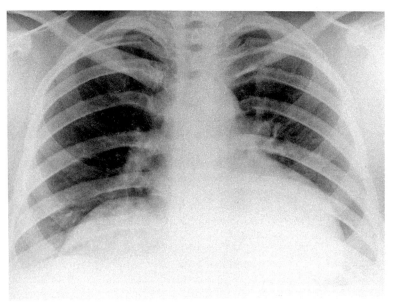

Figure Q40.1

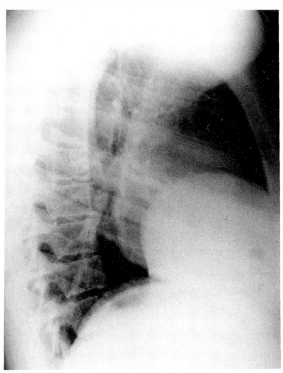

Figure Q40.2

and left upper chest. There was no past medical history of note and, in particular, she denied any previous respiratory symptoms. Examination revealed obvious discomfort on abducting the arm but a full range of shoulder movement was demonstrated. Inspection and palpation of the chest wall revealed no abnormality. The patient was moderately overweight, the apex beat was impalpable and the heart sounds faint, but examination of the chest was otherwise normal.

X-rays of the left humerus showed no bony injury, but the casualty officer was taken aback by the appearances of the chest X-ray. The postero-anterior and right lateral view radiographs are illustrated in Figures Q40.1 and Q40.2, respectively. After being seen, however, by the surgical registrar it was suggested that the girl was allowed home and given an early outpatient appointment for the chest clinic. When seen two weeks later, she was asymptomatic. A thoracic CT scan (Figure Q40.3) was carried out.

54

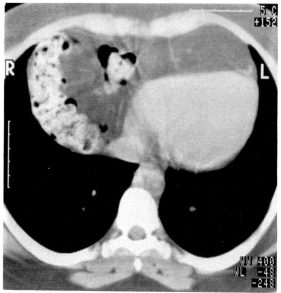
Figure Q40.3

Questions

1. Describe the CT abnormality.
2. What is the diagnosis?

Case 41

On each occasion she had seen her general practitioner Mrs Fergusson, a 28-year-old housewife, had been given the distinct impression that 'it was all in her mind'. She had first visited the surgery five months before, complaining of tiredness and shortness of breath especially when hurrying and when carrying heavy shopping. Her general practitioner had found no abnormal physical signs and had been inclined to attribute her symptoms to a weight problem. Three months later Mrs Fergusson attended again complaining of increased lethargy and breathlessness. She was tearful and depressed and she was prescribed an

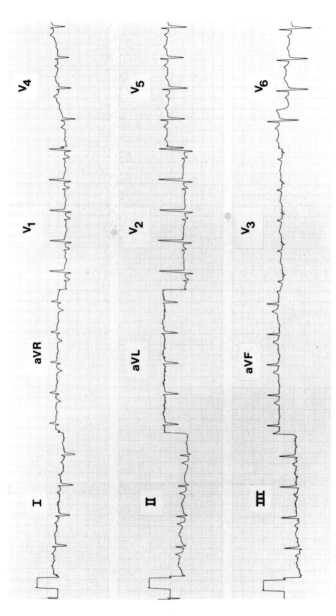

Figure Q41.1

antidepressant. Six weeks later specialist referral was arranged when, having noted no improvement, she reattended the surgery complaining that she felt totally exhausted. The least exertion made her breathless and often lightheaded.

By the time she was seen in outpatients Mrs Fergusson's lethargy and breathlessness had been present for about six months. In the previous four weeks she had also been aware of intermittent central chest discomfort which she had taken to be indigestion but which usually followed exertion. She denied any history of cough, sputum or haemoptysis. She appeared to be happily married with two children (aged 4 and 6 years). She had been a regular smoker of 5–10 cigarettes a day for 8 years. There was a history of a left lower limb deep venous thrombosis complicating her first pregnancy but there was no other past medical history of note.

On examination Mrs Fergusson was mildly overweight and peripherally cyanosed. The pulse was regular and of low volume, rate 100 beats/min, blood pressure 96/54. The apex beat was not displaced. Chest auscultation revealed a loud P_2 and a right atrial fourth sound. There were no murmurs and the lung fields were clear with no adventitious sounds. There were no abnormal abdominal or CNS findings. A chest film showed a normal heart size and silhouette, clear lung fields and some prominence of the main pulmonary arteries. The ECG is reproduced in Figure Q41.1. Pulmonary function tests showed normal lung volumes with only slight impairment of total carbon monoxide gas transfer. A ventilation/perfusion lung scan showed no abnormality.

Questions

1. Describe the ECG abnormalities.
2. What is the probable clinical diagnosis?
3. What is the outlook?

Case 42

Mr James Milligan, a 60-year-old retired miner, was admitted to hospital with one week's history of increasing breathlessness and malaise. For years he had suffered a cough which, most mornings, was productive of small amounts of mucoid sputum. In the previous week, however, his sputum had increased in amount and had become green in colour. He had been quite disabled for some months with an effort tolerance normally limited to about 100 metres on the flat, but in the 24 hours prior to admission to hospital he had become dyspnoeic on minimal exertion and was unable to climb a flight of stairs without stopping several times. There was no history of haemoptysis or ankle swelling. He denied any recent dyspepsia or abdominal pain.

In the past Mr Milligan had been noted for his heavy alcohol consumption and he had been hospitalized on several occasions in latter years on account of alcohol abuse. He admitted to drinking about a quarter of a bottle of whisky per day. Five years before he had suffered an episode of pancreatitis and twelve months earlier an acute duodenal ulcer had been diagnosed on a barium meal. He was a regular smoker of about 30 cigarettes a day.

On examination, he was tachypnoeic and centrally cyanosed with a low grade pyrexia and a regular tachycardia of 110 beats/min. The blood pressure was 155/98. The chest showed an increased antero-posterior diameter, expansion was symmetrically reduced and the percussion note was generally hyper-resonant. Expiration was prolonged. Auscultation revealed marked generalized reduction in the intensity of breath sounds, bilateral inspiratory and expiratory wheeze and coarse crackles localized to the left base. The jugular venous pressure was raised only during expiration and there was no ankle oedema. Abdominal examination was normal. A chest X-ray was reported as showing a normal heart size and silhouette with 'emphysematous lung fields', but no focal lung lesion.

Over the next 24 hours obvious clinical improvement followed treatment with nebulized salbutamol, amoxycillin, continuous 24% oxygen and chest physiotherapy. However two days after admission Mr Milligan's condition rapidly deteriorated. After returning from the bathroom he suddenly collapsed complaining of extreme breathlessness and poorly localized left-sided chest pain. Mr Milligan was alert, anxious and perspiring freely. He was deeply cyanosed with a small volume pulse, rate 120 beats/min and a blood pressure of 100/80. On auscultation wheeze was now most readily audible on the right side. There was no abdominal tenderness and bowel sounds were present. The ECG was unchanged from that recorded upon admission.

Questions

1. What is the most likely cause of Mr Milligan's sudden deterioration?
2. What is the most important aspect of Mr Milligan's immediate management?

Case 43

For three weeks Mrs Finney, a 23-year-old housewife, had been getting steadily worse. She had seen her general practitioner for the first time about a week before complaining of breathlessness which had developed over the previous fortnight. This had been associated with feverishness and cough productive of scanty clear sputum. A viral illness was suspected but an antibiotic (amoxycillin) was prescribed nevertheless. Over the course of the next week Mrs Finney noted increasing malaise and she became progressively more short of breath to the point where she was unable to carry out any housework. Upon being called to the house the general practitioner found his patient living in cramped accomodation in a dirty tenement block. She was sitting propped up in bed alert and orientated, but tachypnoeic and centrally cyanosed with a tachycardia of 126 beats/min and a low grade pyrexia (37.8°C). There was no finger clubbing. She was peripherally well perfused with a blood pressure of 110/60. Chest auscultation revealed widespread, high-pitched inspiratory crackles throughout both lung fields as the only abnormality. The jugular venous pressure was normal and there was no dependent oedema. Immediate hospital admission was arranged.

When seen on the acute medical ward a short time later, there was little to add to the general practitioner's history and physical findings. Mrs Finney was in fact a poor and rather reluctant historian. Over the previous week her cough had been essentially non-productive. She denied having had any chest pain and gave no past medical history of note. She was a lifelong non-smoker. Her husband worked in the shipyards and was a keen pigeon-fancier.

The haemoglobin was 11.4 g/dl, white blood count 14.4×10^9/l with a mild neutrophilia and the ESR 76 mm/h. Arterial blood gases (on air) gave a Pao_2 of 4.40 kPa and a $Paco_2$ of 2.40 kPa, pH 7.38.

The chest X-ray showed diffuse, bilateral and predominantly nodular shadowing. Her extremely scanty mucoid sputum yielded no significant growth. Subsequently, a Mantoux test using 1/100 tuberculin gave no induration at 48 hours. Blood cultures were negative and the first set of viral titres gave negative results for the normally tested respiratory pathogens: influenza A, influenza B, parainfluenza, adenovirus, *Coxiella burnetti, Mycoplasma pneumoniae* and *Chlamydia psittaci.*

Questions

1. What diagnosis do you suspect?
2. Suggest one confirmatory investigation.

Case 44

Apart from treatment for genitourinary tuberculosis at the age of 28 Mrs Sullivan had previously enjoyed excellent health. Now, having just turned 60, it seemed she was never away from the doctor's surgery. For some four to five years she had complained of pain principally affecting the wrists and metacarpophalangeal joints of both hands. Over a similar period she had suffered troublesome heartburn and recently she had noticed some difficulty with swallowing solid food. She had also complained of painful fingers which turned blue in the cold and which her doctor had attributed to 'poor circulation'. The general practitioner finally decided on hospital referral when she presented, yet again, this time with a new complaint of breathlessness on exertion and an associated dry cough which had developed over the previous 12 months.

Mrs Sullivan was an ex-smoker of 15 years duration. Her 62-year-old brother was diabetic and her mother had suffered from rheumatoid arthritis. Apart from an antacid she took no regular medication. Physical examination revealed a few scattered facial telangiectases. There was no clear clinical indication of arthropathy. There were bilateral, basal late inspiratory lung crackles. The haemoglobin was 13.2 g/dl, white blood cell count 8.0 × 10^9/l and ESR 7 mm/h. The serum was negative for rheumatoid factor but positive for antinuclear factor at a titre of

1:64. Radiographs of the hands showed erosive changes affecting the first carpo-metacarpal joints but were otherwise normal. A barium meal examination showed some dilatation of the lower half of the oesophagus, with loss of normal peristalsis and stasis of barium. The chest X-ray showed bilateral reticulo-nodular shadowing with a honeycomb pattern predominantly affecting the lower zones. Pulmonary function tests revealed a moderately severe restrictive ventilatory defect with significant impairment of gas transfer.

Questions

1. What is the most likely clinical diagnosis?
2. What is the treatment?
3. What is the prognosis?

Case 45

Mr John Clements, a 26-year-old store manager had suffered with asthma as a child but he had had less trouble in adult life. He generally became wheezy after upper respiratory infections and in association with exercise, but he used a salbutamol inhaler – his sole treatment – only occasionally. He was a lifelong non-smoker.

He had been well until two weeks before when, after a 'cold', he developed a cough productive of yellow sputum. Breathlessness and wheeze increased but he was able to continue at work and he waited a full week before attending the local surgery. The general practitioner found his chest to be clear and a week's course of amoxycillin was prescribed.

Over the next week his sputum became clear but he continued to suffer from a dry cough, especially at night. His breathlessness also increased and his chest felt particularly 'tight' in the mornings. As long as he took his time, he managed his work without too much difficulty but he was having to use his inhaler much more often and its effect seemed to wear off more quickly than usual. By the end of the week he was persistently short of breath and on the Friday evening Mr Clements was glad to get home. He felt a little easier after his evening meal. However, after retiring to bed he was awoken at 2.00 a.m. by severe shortness of breath. His inhaler afforded him no relief.

After some difficulty in getting through Mrs Clements succeeded in calling out the deputizing doctor who was on call. The patient was found to be tachypnoeic with a tachycardia of 130 beats/min. He was able to hold a conversation only with difficulty. Some improvement followed intravenous administration of aminophylline and, satisfied with this, the 'emergency doctor' left, advising Mr Clements to attend the surgery after the weekend. However, Mr Clements' improvement was only temporary. He was unable to return to sleep and by the following morning he was worse than ever. After his wife's emergency call Mr Clements was immediately tranferred to hospital, receiving continuous 24% oxygen during transit.

On arrival Mr Clements was distressed, agitated and centrally cyanosed with a sinus tachycardia of 160 beats/min and marked arterial paradox. Expiration was markedly prolonged. In the chest, breath sounds were greatly diminished and no adventitious sounds were audible. The peak flow rate was unrecordable. Arterial blood gases showed a Pa_{O_2} of 5.60 kPa with a Pa_{CO_2} of 7.19 kPa. A chest film showed marked hyperinflation with no focal abnormality. The ECG showed marked right heart strain. Treatment with nebulized salbutamol and ipratropium, an aminophylline infusion and continued oxygen therapy resulted in no clinical improvement. Forty minutes after admission the Pa_{CO_2} had climbed to 9.33 kPa.

Questions

1. What treatment is now required?
2. Suggest three aspects of Mr Clement's management which might have been improved.

Case 46

Mr Hamish Lennox, a 57-year-old shopkeeper, had always enjoyed good health but in the three days prior to his hospital admission he had become acutely unwell. Mr Lennox was unable to give a coherent history but his wife related that, at the outset, he had complained of an unproductive cough and a dull frontal headache. Within 24 hours he had developed mild abdominal discomfort associated with watery diarrhoea. Mrs Lennox became increasingly concerned about her husband when, in the day prior to admission, she noted that he was intermittently confused with a staggering gait and slurred speech. There was no previous history of respiratory disease and Mr Lennox had never smoked cigarettes. He was, however, a heavy drinker of about half a bottle of whisky a day.

On examination at the time of admission, he was tachypnoeic, pyrexial (40°C), mildly icteric and confused. The cardiac rhythm was regular, rate 124 beats/min, blood pressure 184/105. The heart sounds were normal with a soft ejection murmur at the left sternal edge. Extensive coarse crackles were audible throughout the left lung field. Abdominal examination was normal. Mr Lennox co-operated poorly with neurological testing and co-ordination was difficult to assess. However, marked lateral nystagmus was noted.

Urinalysis showed haematuria and proteinuria. The haemoglobin was 12.7 g/dl, white blood count 12.0×10^9/l with a lymphopenia, ESR 58 mm/h. His electrolytes were normal apart from a sodium of 132 mmol/l and hypophosphataemia (0.5 mmol/l). Liver function tests gave the following results: bilirubin 84 μmol/l, albumin 33 g/l, alkaline phosphatase 184 IU/l, AST 128 IU/l, ALT 145 IU/l. The LDH was 703 IU/l and the CK 202 IU/l. Arterial blood gases breathing air showed mild arterial hypoxaemia (Pa_{O_2} 9.90 kPa) with a Pa_{CO_2} of 3.40 kPa. Sputum was unobtainable and blood cultures were sterile. A chest X-ray showed left lower lobe consolidation.

Questions

1. What is the most likely diagnosis?
2. What specific therapy is indicated?

Case 47

For some years before he retired Mr McCulloch had been short of breath on exertion. This had gradually progressed in severity, especially over the previous four years, such that now, at the age of

74, his effort tolerance was limited to about 200 metres on the level and he was breathless on climbing one flight of stairs. He admitted to coughing small amounts of clear spit on most days for as long as he could remember. There was no history of haemoptysis. Despite a normal appetite he had lost about two stones in weight, although this had been a gradual development over the previous two to three years. Mr McCulloch denied any joint or gastrointestinal symptoms.

He had retired from the mines at the age of 65 having worked at the coalface for about 40 years. A chest X-ray at this time had been reported as showing small bilateral nodular opacities but he was refused a pension. He had smoked about 15 cigarettes a day for most of his days. Four years before he had undergone a bowel resection and colostomy for carcinoma of the colon.

On examination, Mr McCulloch appeared thin and frail. There was no evident finger clubbing or lymphadenopathy. He was apyrexial. The cardiac rhythm was regular, rate 80 beats/min, blood pressure 166/82. The chest showed an increased antero-posterior diameter with hyper-resonant percussion note,

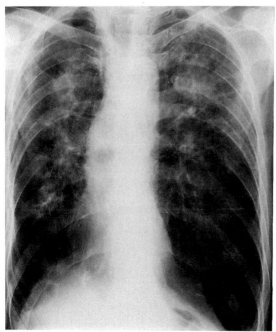

Figure Q47.1

diminished hepatic dullness to percussion, expiratory wheeze and coarse early inspiratory lung crackles. Abdominal examination revealed a functioning colostomy and no other specific abnormality. The haemoglobin was 16.0 g/dl, white blood count 6.1 × 10^9/l, ESR 9 mm/h. Plasma electrolytes and liver function tests were within normal limits. The chest X-ray is shown in Figure Q47.1 and Mr McCulloch's lung function results are reproduced in Table Q47.1.

Table Q47.1   Results of lung function tests*

	Predicted	Actual	% Predicted
FEV$_1$	2.32	0.8 (0.8)**	34.4
FVC	3.46	2.15 (2.16)**	62.1
FEV/FVC%	63.4	40.0	63.0
FRC	4.5	4.6	102
RV	2.28	3.99	175
TLC	6.00	5.91	98.5
RV/TLC%	42.0	67.5	160
TLCO	7.29	2.88	39.4
KCO	3.62	0.59	48.3

* For abbreviations and units, see page x.
** Results after inhaled bronchodilator.

Questions

1. Describe the abnormalities of pulmonary function.
2. What is the most likely cause for the abnormal radiographic shadowing?

Case 48

Mrs Anne Warren, a 66-year-old housewife, was admitted for investigation with a six-month history of lethargy, malaise and progressive weight loss of about two stones. For about two weeks she claimed she had felt exhausted and she had been more or less bed bound. For two days she had also been aware of some sharp pain on breathing in the right lower chest posteriorly. Despite her previous smoking habit (10–15 cigarettes a day for 40 years) Mrs Warren denied any history of cough, sputum or haemoptysis.

There was a past history of cholecystectomy ten years before, angina of effort of six years' duration and myocardial infarction, from which she had made an uneventful recovery 12 months previously. Her Current medication consisted of atenolol (100 mg daily) and glyceryl trinitrate which she seldom used.

Despite the fact that she had lost weight Mrs Warren was markedly obese. She appeared pale and unwell. Firm, non-tender lymphadenopathy was noted in the superficial and deep cervical chains bilaterally and in both axillae. She was mildly pyrexial (37.5°C). The cardiac rhythm was regular at 88 beats/min, blood pressure 152/90. Cardiac and chest auscultation revealed nothing abnormal. Abdominal examination disclosed moderate spleno-megaly as the only abnormality. There was slight pitting oedema of the left ankle.

Routine investigations gave the following results: haemoglobin 9.6 g/dl, white blood count 5.3 × 10^9/l, platelets 150 × 10^9/l, ESR 105 mm/h. Plasma electrolytes and biochemical tests of liver function were normal except for hypoalbuminaemia (28 g/l). The total serum globulin was elevated at 39 g/l. An ECG showed sinus rhythm with left axis deviation and evidence of an old inferior myocardial infarction. The chest X-ray showed bilateral hilar and right-sided paratracheal lymphadenopathy. There was also mild cardiomegaly with a small area of linear atelectasis at the right base and slight elevation of the right hemidiaphragm. Underlying malignancy was strongly suspected, and lymph node biopsy and bone marrow examination were arranged.

However, 24 hours following admisssion, the medical SHO was called to see Mrs Warren whose condition had deteriorated abruptly. She was found to be mentally obtunded, tachypnoeic and centrally cyanosed despite 40% oxygen via a facemask. There was a tachycardia of 160 beats/min with poor peripheral perfusion and she was markedly hypotensive (80/40). The jugular venous pressure was elevated and a gallop rhythm was heard. The chest was clear on auscultation. An ECG showed T wave inversion in leads V1–V6 as the only new abnormality. A chest X-ray was unchanged compared with that 24 hours earlier.

Questions

1. What is the likely cause of Mrs Warren's deterioration?
2. What specific treatment is indicated?

Case 49

Mrs Elsie Stephens, a 34-year-old typist, had seen her general practitioner on no fewer than six occasions over the previous 18 months and she was beginning to feel a fraud. Throughout the whole period she had felt generally unwell and she had tired easily, but her main concern was chest pain. At first this had been intermittent but, latterly, it had been more or less constant; an aching central chest discomfort which was worse when she lay flat, sometimes with sharp pain on deep inspiration. There had never been any abnormal physical signs when she had attended the surgery and her chest pain was thought to have been non-specific. Hospital referral was arranged, however, when Mrs Stephens attended on the sixth occasion still complaining of the same symptoms.

On going over the history in outpatients, Mrs Stephens also admitted to two episodes of 'pleurisy' for which she had received antibiotic therapy. The first had been around the time she began to feel unwell and the most recent episode about six months prior to her clinic attendance. She denied any history of cough or haemoptysis but she had been aware of breathlessness in the previous six months especially when lying flat. Mrs Stephens had also suffered intermittent discomfort and stiffness affecting the wrists and fingers of both hands, but this had been mild and she had not thought to mention it to her general practitioner. She had been asthmatic up to the age of fourteen at which time her symptoms appeared to leave her. There was a history of depressive illness three years before and she admitted that she still felt down from time to time. She was a recent ex-smoker of 10 cigarettes a day.

On examination, Mrs Stephens appeared anxious with a tachycardia of 110 beats/min. She was apyrexial. The blood pressure was 110/65. The heart sounds were normal but a pericardial friction rub was faintly audible. The chest was clear. There was no evidence of any skin eruption and no indication of joint inflammation but patchy alopecia was noted.

The haemoglobin was 10.3 g/dl, white blood count 12.8×10^9/l, ESR 124 mm/h. The blood film showed mild anisocytosis as the only abnormality. Routine urinalysis, plasma electrolytes and liver function tests were all normal. Serum rheumatoid factor was negative. The chest X-ray showed a moderate increase in the cardiac transverse diameter with a flask-shaped cardiac silhouette. Both hemidiaphragms were markedly elevated with areas of 'linear atelectasis' at both bases but otherwise clear lung fields. Lung function tests revealed a moderate restrictive ventilatory defect with reduced total gas transfer but with a normal K_{CO}.

Questions

1. What is the most likely clinical diagnosis?
2. What is the explanation for the radiographic abnormalities?

Case 50

Mr Robert Syme, a 50-year-old postman, had been perfectly well until one week before. His illness had started abruptly with headache, malaise and chills followed within 24 hours by cough and right-sided pleuritic chest pain. There was no history of previous respiratory illness but Mr Syme had been a regular smoker of 30 cigarettes a day. On being called to the house the general practitioner found his patient to be pyrexial (38.5°C) with obvious signs of consolidation at the right base posteriorly. A right lower lobe pneumonia was diagnosed and amoxycillin prescibed. Mr Syme was advised to maintain a higher than normal fluid intake and he was given sublingual buprenorphine for pain relief.

At the outset his cough was unproductive but over the course of the next few days he produced moderate amounts of slightly bloodstained mucopurulent sputum. After three days his pain was less and his temperature was 37.4°C. However, he remained anorectic and he continued to feel unwell. His general practitioner elected to review progress once again at the end of the week. At this stage, seven days after the onset of his illness, Mr Syme was no better and hospital admission was requested.

On arrival he remained pyrexial (38.0°C) with a tachycardia of 110 beats/min, blood pressure 120/70. The heart sounds were normal with no added sounds or murmurs. Examination of the chest revealed reduced movement on the right side. There was marked dullness to percussion posteriorly in the right middle and lower zones and reduction in the intensity of breath sounds in the same distribution. Abdominal examination was normal.

The haemoglobin was 11.3 g/dl, white blood count 25.1 × 10⁹/l with a neutrophilia. Plasma electrolytes were normal. The serum albumin was 25 g/l and globulin 43 g/l. The chest X-ray showed extensive hazy shadowing in the right middle and lower zones. A lateral view revealed a large homogeneous D-shaped shadow lying posteriorly, extending from the diaphragm to the level of the fourth thoracic vertebra.

Questions

1. Why did Mr Syme fail to respond to antibiotic therapy?
2. What therapeutic alternatives are available now?

Answers and Discussions

Case 1

Answers

1. Restrictive ventilatory defect of moderate severity with impairment of gas transfer.
2. (a) Lymphangitis carcinomatosa
   (b) Pulmonary asbestosis
   (c) Fibrosing alveolitis
3. (a) Diagnostic bronchoalveolar lavage
   (b) Lung biopsy

Although Mr Thompson clearly has angina of effort and there is a family history of ischaemic heart disease, his symptoms are unlikely to have a cardiac cause. The radiographic appearances are consistent with pulmonary oedema, but the heart size and silhouette are within normal limits, there are no clinical features of cardiac failure and there are no physical or ECG signs of cardiac abnormality. The combination of wheeze, progressive dyspnoea and previous smoking habit suggests the possibility of chronic obstructive lung disease. The patient's troublesome symptoms are of only four weeks duration, however, and there are no clinical features to suggest an infective exacerbation. Furthermore, pulmonary function tests show restriction of lung volumes and no evidence of airflow obstruction.

The patient's occupation will inevitably have brought him into contact with asbestos. Radiographic evidence of pleural thickening and pleural calcification is in keeping with previous asbestos exposure and lung function results are certainly consistent with diffuse pulmonary fibrosis. Asbestosis normally presents with an insidious onset and progression of breathlessness. It may present subacutely when complicated by bronchial carcinoma, the cause of death in roughly half of all asbestosis patients, but there is little to suggest this diagnosis. Finger clubbing accompanies asbestosis in about 50% of cases, but is absent here. Similarly, the presence of bilateral basal late inspiratory crackles typifies about 60% of cases of asbestosis. They may be difficult or even impossible to hear when there is substantial, bilateral pleural thickening, but this does not apply to the present case and the absence of basal crackles is further evidence against a diagnosis of asbestosis. These two physical signs (finger clubbing and basal lung crackles) would also be expected in the majority of cases of cryptogenic fibrosing alveolitis. In fact, lung biopsy showed widespread permeation of lymphatic channels by poorly differentiated adenocarcinoma.

Disseminated tumour involvement affecting lymphatic or vascular spaces within the lungs is a common cause of widespread radiographic lung shadowing and this possibility must often be considered in the differential diagnosis of diffuse 'interstitial' lung disease. There are commonly no abnormal physical signs and finger clubbing in particular is unusual. The most characteristic X-ray abnormalities consist of enlarged hilar lymph nodes with radiating long hair-line shadows (Kerley's A lines), representing infiltrated lymphatics, extending from the hilar regions to the lung periphery. Linear shadows are frequently inconspicuous, however. The chest radiograph often shows a more nodular appearance and the extent of lymphatic involvement may only be appreciated in tissue sections.

This patient posed an additional diagnostic problem. The primary tumour is clinically occult in as many as 5–10% of all patients with histologically confirmed metastatic cancer and there is commonly some confusion as to how intensively the primary should be sought. In general, such patients are often over investigated. It is common but frequently mistaken to assume that diagnosing the primary will inevitably improve the prospects of successful treatment. Equally, it is not necessarily the case that the harder the primary is sought, the more likely it is to be found. In fact, the primary remains undetected even at postmortem in up to 20% of tumours of unknown origin. Furthermore, the outlook for the majority of these patients is very poor, with a median survival in most series limited to about three months. Once a tissue diagnosis has been established therefore, further investigations should be minimized and restricted to those aimed at identifying tumours which are potentially curable or for which particularly effective treatment is available.

Metastatic adenocarcinoma from any primary site is unlikely to be curable but specific and effective treatments are available for breast, thyroid, ovarian and prostatic cancers, all of which must be carefully excluded in a patient presenting with the clinical picture described in this case. Immuno-cytochemical staining techniques applied to the original biopsy material (e.g. measurement of cytoplasmic steroid receptors in the case of breast cancer, staining with antibodies to thyroglobulin or prostate-specific acid phosphatase) may be of great value in identifying these tumour types. Mr Robertson was found to have a greatly raised serum prostatic acid phosphatase and the diagnosis of prostatic carcinoma was confirmed by prostatic biopsy.

Further reading

STEWART, J. F., TATTERSALL, M. H. N., WOODS, R. L. and FOX, R. M. (1979). Unknown primary adenocarcinoma: incidence of over investigation and natural history. *British Medical Journal,* **1,** 1530.

Case 2

Answers

1. Pulmonary tuberculosis
2. (a) Bronchial carcinoma
   (b) Lung abscess

The differential diagnosis is that of haemoptysis in a patient with a solitary intrapulmonary cavity. The diagnoses listed above represent the three commonest causes of a lung cavity and all commonly give rise to haemoptysis. Repeated small haemoptyses occurring on a regular, daily basis over a period of one or more weeks .is characteristic of bronchial carcinoma, but all three conditions may present with a large or even massive (greater than 500 ml/24 h) haemoptysis.

In this case a definite diagnosis of tuberculosis was established from positive sputum cultures several weeks after the patient's presentation, but the diagnosis was strongly suspected on clinical grounds and antituberculous therapy was initiated on this basis. Thus, the presence of radiological evidence (right mid-zone and right hilar calcification) of previous primary tuberculosis lends support to the diagnosis. The diagnostic value of the tuberculin test is limited in this and other countries where there is widespread use of BCG vaccination as a method of tuberculosis control. However, a strongly positive test as in the present case, whilst in itself non-diagnostic, makes tuberculosis more likely; a weak positive or negative reaction reduces the likelihood of tuberculosis, but does not exclude this diagnosis. The patient's background of alcoholism is also consistent with the clinical diagnosis. The relatively high incidence of tuberculosis among alcoholics is well recognized. This may relate, at least in part, to the commonly associated malnutrition but a direct immunosuppressant effect of alcohol and other ill-understood factors are probably implicated.

Lung abscess due to pyogenic organisms usually renders the patient more acutely ill than is the case with tuberculosis. The clinical history is usually shorter and the patient more highly febrile with a prominent neutrophil leucocytosis. A discharging lung abscess is associated with frankly purulent sputum from which the causative organism is usually readily isolated.

Sputum is usually positive on direct smear in cases of tuberculous cavitation, but this is by no means always the case. When the patient is direct smear negative, especially in cases where there is an isolated cavity, the differential diagnosis from bronchial carcinoma is made more difficult. In these circumstances, a normal bronchoscopy helps to exclude the possibility of a lung abscess arising distal to an obstructing neoplasm, but does not exclude a more peripheral, cavitating tumour beyond bronchoscopic range. Bacteriological and cytological examination of bronchial aspirate and fluoroscopically-guided brush biopsies may be helpful. Certain radiological features may help to differentiate neoplastic and tuberculous cavities, but total reliance upon these features is unwise. A typical tuberculous cavity occupies the posterior segment of an upper lobe or the apical segment of a lower lobe. The presence of adjacent, 'satellite' shadows and calcification, best seen in tomograms, is also suggestive of tuberculosis. By contrast a neoplastic cavity is more likely to be situated anteriorly and, typically, tomography shows an eccentric cavity with a thick, irregular wall. Common associated features include enlargement of draining lymph nodes, an irregular outer margin with radiating linear shadows ('sunburst' appearance), and evidence of bone erosion.

Where a definite diagnosis cannot be made, particularly when tuberculosis appears less likely on clinical grounds, a diagnostic thoracotomy may be wiser than the alternative course of action where thoracotomy is deferred until tuberculosis cultures are

Table A2.1   Causes of intrapulmonary cavities

Infective

Tuberculosis
Primary and embolic (pyaemic) lung abscesses
Lung abscess complicating bronchial obstruction e.g. secondary to
    bronchial carcinoma
    inhaled foreign body
Septic pulmonary infarct
Necrotizing pneumonia e.g. secondary to
    pyogenic, especially staphylococcal infection
    -amoebic infection
Mycetoma and other fungal infections
Paragonimiasis
Secondarily infected cysts or bullae
Ruptured hydatid cyst

Neoplastic

Primary bronchial carcinoma
Pulmonary metastases
Hodgkin's disease

Developmental

Bronchogenic cyst
Sequestrated lung segment
Polycystic lobe

Miscellaneous lesions causing focal lung necrosis

Wegener's granulomatosis
Necrotic rheumatoid nodule
Pulmonary infarction
Pneumoconiosis (necrosis in areas of PMF)

available or until the response to antituberculous therapy has been assessed. The fact that bronchial carcinoma and tuberculosis may co-exist further confounds the diagnosis in a small proportion of cases and this possibility must be borne in mind. In addition to the differential diagnosis already discussed, it should be noted that a wide diversity of diseases may produce intrapulmonary cavitation and these too must be considered in the appropriate clinical context (Table A2.1).

Case 3

Answers

1. Subphrenic abscess
2. (a) Diaphragmatic screening
   (b) Upper abdominal ultrasound
   (c) Upper abdominal computed tomography (CT)

This patient's clinic attendences in 1977 and again in 1983 were fairly clearly related to anxiety, but in 1984 it might appear that Mrs Warren's fear of 'cancer' was well founded. Progressive weight loss, haemoptysis and finger clubbing in a middle-aged smoker are most certainly suggestive of bronchial carcinoma. However, the patient's illness is also characterized by a recurrent pyrexia and cough with persistently purulent sputum, whilst bronchoscopy showed evidence of only inflammatory changes. Bronchiectasis, which might be considered in the differential diagnosis, is generally not associated with major systemic upset and would be unlikely to present for the first time in a woman of 52. The clinical picture strongly suggests an untreated source of infection producing recurrent pneumonitis. The presence of a tender upper abdominal mass and the fact that Mrs Warren's clinical deterioration followed abdominal surgery point to the possibility of a subphrenic abscess.

An upper abdominal abscess most commonly arises as a complication of abdominal surgery, either gastric or biliary surgery being implicated in the majority of cases. Early recognition is of paramount importance. Delayed diagnosis is associated with an increased mortality rate which approaches 25% even with surgical drainage. Abscesses may be located beneath the diaphragm or, alternatively, in the subhepatic space or the lesser sac. Both upper abdominal quadrants are affected with approximately equal frequency. The usual causative organisms include coliforms, streptococci and gas-producing anaerobes.

Clinical evidence of systemic infection is usually apparent and the diagnosis is generally obvious in the appropriate clinical setting. Diagnosis is less straightforward when some time has elapsed following the initial predisposing event or when the patient presents with thoracic complications without evidence of abdominal disease. As many as 80% of patients develop a pleural effusion. This is normally a sterile exudate containing abundant polymorphs, but it may become an empyema, especially if diagnosis and treatment are delayed. The inflammatory process may also spread to the adjacent lung resulting in a basal pneumonia. The plain chest X-ray is therefore an important diagnostic aid as it will often show one or more of the following features: ipsilateral pleural fluid, basal consolidation or elevation of the diaphragm on the affected side. Occasionally, when the abscess is secondary to gas-forming organisms or when it has resulted from a ruptured viscus, there is an air-fluid level below the diaphragm in the upright view.

The diagnosis may be facilitated by a variety of imaging procedures. Elevation and fixation of the diaphragm may be demonstrable by simple fluoroscopy, but frequently the level and movement of the diaphragm are obscured by pleural fluid and screening is generally only of limited value. Abdominal ultrasound and CT scanning offer the most effective means of identifying and localizing upper abdominal abscesses. The latter is particularly effective for identifying a lesion in the left upper quadrant where the normal gastric air-fluid level and gas in the splenic flexure render diagnosis by ultrasound more difficult.

Case 4

Answers

1. Histiocytosis-X (eosinophilic granuloma)
2. (a) Lung biopsy; light microscopy can be diagnostic but electron microscopy will often show pathognomonic ultrastructural, cytoplasmic complexes (Birbeck granules) within abnormal histiocytes
   (b) Skeletal survey for lytic bone lesions
   (c) Water deprivation test (for diagnosis of associated diabetes insipidus)

Pneumothoraces may be *spontaneous* (secondary to pulmonary or pleural abnormality), *artificial* (following the deliberate introduction of air into the pleural cavity) or *traumatic* in aetiology. Most spontaneous pneumothoraces are diagnosed in young adult males when the vast majority of cases result from the rupture of an apical subpleural 'bleb' arising from a chance congenital weakness in the alveolar wall. In older patients spontaneous pneumothorax most often arises as a complication of chronic bronchitis and emphysema. Less commonly, the condition complicates a variety of 'focal' (e.g. ruptured congenital cyst, ruptured tuberculous cavity, ruptured tension cyst in staphylococcal pneumonia or bronchial carcinoma) and 'diffuse' lung disorders (e.g. bronchial asthma, pneumoconiosis, sarcoidosis, systemic sclerosis and other causes of interstitial pulmonary fibrosis). In the case of interstitial lung disorders pneumothorax is generally a feature of advanced disease when widespread architectural distortion leads to rupture of subpleural cysts.

Lung involvement in certain rare conditions (*histiocytosis-X, tuberous sclerosis, lymphangioleiomyomatosis* and neurofibromatosis) is characterized by particularly extensive cystic change or 'honeycombing' and pneumothorax is an especially frequent complication. These disorders share similar radiographic features and often show the same distinctive pattern of lung function abnormality (see below), but they present widely divergent clinical and histopathological characteristics. Tuberous sclerosis is associated with characteristic fibrotic changes under the nails (subungual fibromata), in the kidney and brain and most patients are mentally retarded, the condition being inherited as an autosomal recessive. Neurofibromatosis (von Recklinghausen's disease) shows an autosomal dominant pattern of inheritance with characteristic skin changes (café-au-lait pigmentation, shagreen patches) as well as multiple tumours of peripheral nerves. Lymphangioleiomyomatosis is confined to women of childbearing age, the lung changes resulting from widespread hyperplasia of atypical smooth muscle. By contrast, histiocytosis-X (eosinophilic granuloma) is more common in males.

Pulmonary involvement in histiocytosis-X may occur as an isolated phenomenon or in association with disease at other sites. Lytic bone lesions are seen in about 5–10% of cases. Diabetes insipidus, secondary to posterior pituitary involvement, is seen with a similar frequency. Either association, when present, will strongly suggest histiocytosis as the cause of 'honeycomb lungs'. Histologically, the lungs are characterized, in the earlier stages of the disease, by a pleomorphic cellular infiltrate which includes abnormal histiocytes and, frequently, prominent eosinophils. At this stage the chest film usually shows diffuse nodular shadowing. As the disease progresses, disruption of alveolar septa and the development of cysts leads to the more characteristic radiographic appearance of 'honeycombing'. Contrasting functional abnormalities may also be noted, corresponding to the early and later stages of the disease. Thus, the initial pulmonary infiltrate is associated with restriction of lung volumes, impairment of gas transfer and reduced lung compliance. The progressive increase in cystic changes that characterizes the later stages of the disease results in loss of elastic support for the airways, with increased lung compliance and the development of airflow obstruction. The associated impairment of gas transfer results in an pattern of abnormal lung function which resembles that produced by emphysema, a pattern which is common to other causes of 'honeycomb lung' and one which presents a distinct contrast to the functional changes usually seen in pulmonary disorders associated with significant pulmonary fibrosis.

Case 5

Answers

1. An intrabronchial tumour, probably a bronchial adenoma
2. (a) Anterior view tomograms of left lower zone
   (b) Bronchoscopy

A history of variable wheeze and exacerbations associated with respiratory infection strongly suggests bronchial asthma in a non-smoker. In this case, however, the findings on physical examination are not entirely consistent with this diagnosis. Thus, although there is evidence of 'noisy breathing' – a useful sign of airflow obstruction – the patient's spirometry and peak flow rate are within normal limits. At rest, the breath sounds of a healthy subject are inaudible at a distance of just a few centimetres from the mouth. In chronic obstructive bronchitis and asthma turbulent airflow in the lobar and segmental airways causes noisy inspiratory breath sounds and it has been shown that the loudness of the breath sound correlates closely with the severity of airflow obstruction as measured spirometrically. However, there is an important exception to this general rule. This is when turbulent airflow results not from generalized airways obstruction but from a focal area of narrowing affecting one of the larger airways. In these circumstances, a localized wheeze and noisy breathing may be heard when tests of airways function show no abnormality. That this is the explanation here is suggested by the presence of a single left-sided, monophonic wheeze rather than multiple bilateral wheezes of different pitch, a more characteristic finding in bronchial asthma.

The significance of the patient's previous history of left-sided pleurisy may be appreciated after careful inspection of the chest radiographs. The PA film (Figure Q5.1) is virtually normal with only the faint suggestion of an abnormal area of shadowing lying behind

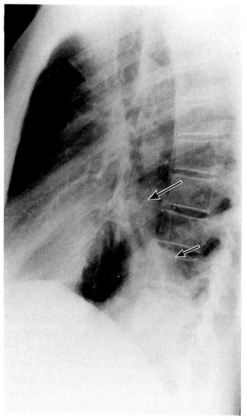

Figure A5.1 Lateral view radiograph corresponding to Figure Q5.2 showing rounded mass (large arrow) and distal left lower lobe consolidation (small arrow)

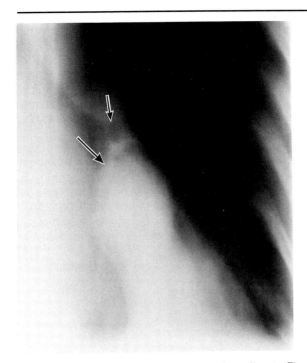

Figure A5.2 Anterior view tomogram corresponding to Figure Q5.1 showing bifurcation of left main stem bronchus; patent upper lobe bronchus (small arrow); lower lobe bronchus (large arrow) obstructed by rounded mass

the heart. The lateral view (Figure A5.1), however, clearly shows a rounded mass (large arrow) with distal consolidation (small arrows) affecting the left lower lobe. The combined clinical and radiographic features suggest the possibility of a lesion causing partial bronchial obstruction and predisposing to recurrent lower respiratory infection. A penetrated radiograph or tomograms could be expected to define the lesion more clearly as in Figure A5.2 which confirms the presence of a well circumscribed opacity occupying the left lower lobe. Bronchoscopy confirmed the presence of a smooth, cherry-like tumour almost completely occluding the left lower lobe bronchus. Bronchial biopsies showed the typical appearances of a 'carcinoid' tumour.

Benign tumours of the respiratory tract are uncommon with an incidence less than (1%) that of primary bronchial carcinomas. Bronchial adenomas are by far the most common benign neoplasms arising within the bronchial tree and two main histological varieties are recognized – 'carcinoid' tumours which account for 80–90% and 'cylindromas'. Although described as benign, adenomas have the potential for malignant transformation (greater in the case of 'cylindromas') which is sometimes evident after several years of non-invasive growth. The majority (about 75%) arise centrally within the bronchial tree, commonly resulting in symptoms due to bronchial obstruction and recurrent haemoptysis. Repeated episodes of infection arising in the same pulmonary segment or lobe over a period of months or years is a particularly characteristic presentation. When the diagnosis is delayed, longstanding bronchial obstruction may give rise to chronic infection with persistently purulent sputum as in bron-chiectasis. A similar clinical picture may be seen following foreign body aspiration which, along with other causes of a localized bronchial obstruction (e.g. bronchial carcinoma, tuberculous bronchostenosis, mucus plugging, intrabronchial metastasis), can be excluded by bronchoscopy.

Bronchial adenomas arising in the lung periphery do not cause bronchial obstruction. The peripheral tumour is usually identified as an incidental finding in the chest radiograph of an asymptomatic patient. The typical radiographic appearance of a rounded, well defined and occasionally lobulated opacity is in no way distinctive and differentiation from other 'coin' lesions requires tissue biopsy. Bronchial carcinoids and cylindromas produce an identical spectrum of clinical and radiological features with the exception that a few carcinoid adenomas will also, though only rarely, produce the classical carcinoid syndrome consisting of attacks of intense facial flushing, bronchospasm, vomiting and diarrhoea. Hormones (serotonin, 5-hydroxy-tryptophan and 5-hydroxyindole-acetic acid) may be produced in sufficient quantity by the primary tumour but, in general, the full-blown carcinoid syndrome suggests considerable tumour bulk and is most commonly therefore confined to the rare instances where malignant metaplasia and metastatic dissemination have occurred.

Further reading

MARKS, C. and MARKS, M. (1977) Bronchial adenoma. A clinicopathological study. *Chest*, **71**, 376.

Case 6

Answers

1. Meigs' syndrome.
2. Probably not. There is sufficient diagnostic information to justify laparotomy as a next step.

As it was originally applied, Meigs' syndrome refers to the association of ascites and pleural effusion(s) with solid benign ovarian tumours. Surgical removal of the pelvic neoplasm is characterized by the complete and permanent disappearance of the effusions. Up to the time of its description by Meigs and Cass (1937), the development of ascites or pleural fluid in a patient with a pelvic mass was regarded as indicative of advanced malignancy. The importance of recognizing the syndrome lies in the potential for surgical cure of what might otherwise be mistaken, on clinical grounds, for inoperable disease.

The tumour most commonly implicated in Meigs' syndrome is the ovarian fibroma but fibroadenomas, cystic ovarian tumours, thecomas, granulosa cell tumours and even uterine fibroleiomyomas may also be responsible. The syndrome may also occur in association with ovarian tumours of low-grade malignancy in the absence of metastatic disease. Its pathogenesis is poorly understood. Secretion from the primary tumour appears to be the source of fluid. Ascites may not be evident on physical examination and, in general, only large tumours are associated with free peritoneal fluid at the time of surgery. A variety of theories have been advanced to explain the pleural abnormality, but it is most likely that fluid passes through defects in the diaphragm.

The pleural effusion is right-sided in about 70% of patients, left-sided in 10% and the remainder have bilateral effusions. Typically the pleural fluid is serous or, occasionally, serosanguinous with a low total white cell count (usually less than 1×10^9/l). Textbook descriptions of Meigs' syndrome commonly refer to it as a cause of hydrothorax (collection of transudate fluid), but in practice the pleural fluid protein is usually above 30 g/l (i.e. an exudate).

About 15% of ovarian fibromas are associated with free ascitic fluid but a much smaller proportion also have a pleural effusion and Meigs' syndrome is undoubtedly therefore a relatively rare occurrence. The concurrent development of ascites and pleural effusion(s) – due to transudation of fluid – is more commonly encountered in association with hypoproteinaemic states (e.g. nephrotic syndrome, hepatic cirrhosis) and congestive cardiac failure and, less commonly, hypothyroidism and constrictive pericarditis. Pleural effusions are a rare complication of drug idiosyncrasy (e.g. associated with nitrofurantoin, methysergide, bromocriptine, procarbazine, methotraxate and dantrolene sodium) and one agent, practolol, has been associated with both pleural and peritoneal changes. Other β-blockers including acebutolol, Mrs Barrie's antianginal medication, have not been implicated however and the clinical illness is quite unlike the distinctive course followed by practolol-induced progressive pleural thickening and sclerosing peritonitis (Marshall *et al.*, 1977). When pleural and ascitic fluid are unequivocally exudates, infection (e.g. tuberculosis) and malignant disease are the most likely diagnoses. In a patient with a pelvic mass Meigs' syndrome should be suspected when pleural and/or peritoneal fluid cytology and pleural biopsies show no evidence of malignancy. The diagnosis is confirmed retrospectively when, following removal of the primary tumour, there is no subsequent recurrence of pleural fluid or ascites.

References

MARSHALL, A. J., ELTRINGHAM, W. K., BARRITT, D. W. *et al.* (1977) Respiratory disease associated with practolol therapy. *Lancet*, **ii**, 1254.
MEIGS, J. V. and CASS, J. W. (1937) Fibroma of the ovary with ascites and hydrothorax. *American Journal of Obstetrics and Gynecology*, **33**, 249.

Case 7

Answers

1. Goodpasture's syndrome.
2. (a) Renal biopsy (following adequate dialysis).
   (b) Serum radioimmunoassay for anti-glomerular basement membrane (anti-GBM) antibody.

Haemoptysis is a common symptom in a wide range of respiratory disorders (inflammatory, infective, neoplastic, embolic) and is also a frequent feature of disease affecting other systems as in cardiac failure and a variety of blood dyscrasias. Profuse bleeding from any site within the lung may cause a transient radiographic abnormality when there is significant aspiration of blood but there is a group of disorders, which includes Goodpasture's syndrome, where diffuse radiographic shadowing complicates bleeding from, specifically, the acinar parts of the lungs. Such alveolar haemorrhage may occur acutely or over a prolonged period and typically gives rise not only to haemoptysis and transient, widespread radiographic shadows but also, in some cases, iron deficiency anaemia.

The clinical diagnosis of alveolar haemorrhage may present difficulties. The severity of haemoptysis is extremely variable and bears little relation to the extent of the radiographic abnormality. At one extreme haemoptysis may be life-threatening while, at the other, widespread microscopic capillary leakage may fail to cause haemoptysis at all. The radiographic picture is also variable, in some cases causing widespread confluent shadows (an 'alveolar filling' pattern) closely resembling pulmonary oedema and in others producing discrete, micronodular ('pinhead') shadows simulating a wide variety of interstitial lung disorders. The diagnosis is supported by the finding of haemosiderin-laden macrophages in the patient's sputum between episodes of haemoptysis. In itself, however, this is a non-specific feature which may be found in any disorder associated with bleeding into the lungs. It is also characteristic of conditions associated with chronically elevated pulmonary venous pressure. Better supportive evidence is provided by measurements of the gas transfer coefficient (K_{co}, i.e. the total carbon monoxide gas transfer – TL_{co} – corrected for effective alveolar volume, V_A). The K_{co} is characteristically elevated in any disorder associated with pulmonary haemorrhage owing to avid carbon monoxide uptake by free haemoglobin for which the test gas has a strong affinity. By contrast, pulmonary oedema results in reduced values for TL_{co} and K_{co}. It is important that values are corrected for blood haemoglobin concentration as the patient is often anaemic. In Goodpasture's syndrome, because of chronic uraemia, the baseline value may be low and a rise in K_{co} may still produce a result within the normal range. Serial measurements are necessary therefore when the K_{co} is often seen to fluctuate in parallel with changing radiographic appearances.

Goodpasture's syndrome refers specifically to the combination of pulmonary haemorrhage and glomerulonephritis caused by antibodies directed against glomerular and alveolar basement membranes. The term should be reserved for cases where there is demonstrable circulating anti-GBM antibody or where the characteristic linear pattern of immunofluorescence (due to deposition of IgG and complement along the glomerular and alveolar basement membranes) is seen in renal or lung biopsies. The association of pulmonary haemorrhage and glomerulonephritis is also seen in certain systemic vasculitides and, rarely, as a complication of therapy with D-penicillamine (Table A7.1). The pathogenetic mechanism is different in these disorders. Renal and pulmonary injury is mediated by circulating immune complexes rather than an autoantibody. Biopsy differentiation from Goodpasture's syndrome is made possible by the presence of electron dense deposits (absent in Goodpasture's syndrome) and a granular, as opposed to a linear, pattern of immunofluoresence. In a proportion of cases immune-complex mediated injury occurs in the absence of multisystem disease.

Table A7.1   Disorders associated with pulmonary haemorrhage and glomerulonephritis

Goodpasture's syndrome
Wegener's granulomatosis
Polyarteritis nodosa (PAN)
Microscopic polyarteritis
Churg-Strauss syndrome
Systemic lupus erythematosus (SLE)
D-penicillamine therapy

Goodpasture's syndrome is predominantly a disease of young adult males (usually aged between 20 and 30 years). Only very occasional cases of spontaneous remission have been recorded and, until relatively recently, the disorder usuaroved fatal with approximately equal numbers of patients dying from massive pulmonary haemorrhage or from renal failure. Most patients present with haemoptysis and only rarely does pulmonary haemorrhage postdate the nephritis. Gross haematuria occurs in 10–40% of patients; when it is absent routine urinalysis will often show a nephritic pattern (red cells with abnormal morphology, red cell and granular casts, proteinuria). The typical renal lesion, a crescentic proliferative glomerulonephritis, is non-specific.

Similar renal histology is seen in polyarteritis nodosa (PAN) and systemic lupus erythematosus (SLE), but electron microscopy and immunofluorescence differentiate (see above). Lung tissue characteristically shows alveolar wall fibrosis, intra-alveolar haemorrhage with haemosiderin-laden macrophages present both in the interstitium and in the alveolar spaces.

The treatment of Goodpasture's syndrome depends upon the removal of circulating antibody by plasmapheresis combined with the prevention of fresh antibody synthesis using immunosuppressants (corticosteroids and cyclophosphamide). When renal disease is not severe (creatinine less than 600 μmol/l) this combined approach may prevent irreversible renal damage and will often control pulmonary haemorrhage. In patients with more severe renal impairment little improvement in renal function can be expected and dialysis will usually be necessary. Despite immunosuppressant therapy dialysis patients remain at risk from major and potentially fatal pulmonary haemorrhage. The suggestion that eliminating the source of antigen, by bilateral nephrectomy, might protect the lungs from further immunological damage has not been borne out in practice.

Further reading

MORGAN, P. G. M. and TURNER-WARWICK, M. (1981) Pulmonary haemosiderosis and pulmonary haemorrhage. *British Journal of Diseases of the Chest*, **75**, 225.

Case 8

Answers

1. Asbestos pleural effusion and pleural thickening.
2. Yes. There may be impairment of lung function and associated disability which is compensatable.
3. Pleural plaque formation, pleural mesothelioma, pulmonary fibrosis (asbestosis), rounded atelecatsis, asbestos granuloma (asbestoma, a solitary fibrotic lesion) and bronchial carcinoma are the other possible pleuropulmonary consequences of asbestos exposure. Peritoneal mesothelioma is a rare but important extrathoracic manifestation; there is probably an increased risk of laryngeal cancer and possibly also certain gastrointestinal cancers as a result of asbestos exposure.

Discrete hyaline and calcified pleural plaques, diffuse pleural thickening and malignant mesothelioma are all well recognized pleural manifestations of asbestos exposure. Pleural effusion is a common presenting feature of mesothelioma but it has become increasingly clear that asbestos exposure may also cause an exudative pleural reaction in the absence of malignant change. Eisenstadt (1964) first mentioned the possible association between asbestos exposure and benign pleural effusion in an insulation worker. More recent observations (Gaensler and Kaplan, 1971) have helped to confirm this association, underlining the need to consider asbestos exposure in the broad differential diagnosis of unexplained pleural effusions. It is believed that asbestos pleural effusions may develop with dust exposures much less than those associated with the development of asbestosis and, for this reason, a particularly careful occupational history may be necessary to elicit what may have been relatively brief, intermittent or remote exposure.

The effusion is generally small or moderate and seldom, if ever, massive. The pleural fluid, a sterile exudate which may be clear or slightly bloodstained, shows no diagnostic features. Diagnosis is based primarily on exclusion and a high level of confidence may only be possible when a period of prolonged observation has failed to suggest an alternative aetiology. Cytological examination of the fluid and pleural needle biopsy are helpful only as means of excluding other possible diagnoses. Open biopsy material showing non-specific pleuritis and thickened pleura with or without rare asbestos bodies lends support to the diagnosis especially if there are also parenchymal changes due to asbestosis, minor degrees of which are a common associated abnormality.

Clinical case histories, like this one, have lent support to the theory (Gaensler and Kaplan, 1971) that such pleural effusions are the aetiological precursor of diffuse pleural thickening. It is probable that because the effusions tend to be relatively small they are usually asymptomatic and often therefore go undetected. In symptomatic cases long-term follow up has shown that the effusions are frequently recurrent, usually bilateral and are associated with pleuritic chest pain which may become persistent.

The functional effects of asbestos pleural disease have been difficult to assess because of the possible additional presence of pulmonary fibrosis and/or airflow obstruction. There is now good evidence, however, that whereas pleural plaques very rarely impair lung function diffuse pleural thickening, especially when it is extensive, is not uncommonly accompanied by a reduction in lung volumes (Britton, 1982) and pleural restriction sufficient to cause disability may necessitate surgical decortication. A distinctive pattern of lung function abnormality may be seen: a restrictive defect accompanied by a reduction in single breath carbon monoxide gas transfer (TL_{co}) but a normal or raised gas transfer coefficient (K_{co}). The K_{co} is obtained by dividing the TL_{co} by the effective alveolar volume, V_A (as determined by helium dilution). A raised value in this setting suggests pleural restriction rather than pulmonary fibrosis as the dominant functional abnormality, with the lungs held rigidly within an abnormal pleura (significant alveolar fibrosis generally leads to a reduction in both the TL_{co} and K_{co}). Table A8.1 shows the other pathological circumstances that are charcteristically associated with a raised K_{co} (see also Case 8).

Table A8.1 Pathological conditions producing a raised K_{co}

Extrapulmonary restriction
  pleural disease
  neuromuscular weakness
  skeletal deformity
Pulmonary haemorrhage*
Bronchial asthma**
Pneumonectomy
Polycythaemia*
Left to right shunts*

* Conditions invariably also associated with a raised TL_{co}
** Conditions occasionally also associated with a raised TL_{co}

References

BRITTON, M. G. (1982) Asbestos pleural disease. *British Journal of Diseases of the Chest*, **76**, 1.

EISENSTADT, H. B. (1964) Asbestos pleurisy. *Diseases of the Chest*, **46**, 78.

GAENSLER, E. A. and KAPLAN, A. I. (1971) Asbestos pleural effusion. *Annals of Internal Medicine*, **74**, 178.

Case 9

Answers

1. Sarcoidosis.
2. Mr Benjamin's skin lesions offered a readily accessible source of biopsy material. One of these revealed a uniform histological picture consisting of an infiltrate of non-caseating epithelioid granulomas, supporting the clinical diagnosis of sarcoidosis.

Although its most important manifestations affect the lungs, sarcoidosis is a multisystem disease characterized by the presence of caseating epithelioid cell tubercles (or their hyalinized remnants) in a number of affected organs or tissues. By convention thoracic sarcoidosis is categorized into four descriptive groups according to the appearance of the chest radiograph:

1. Normal chest X-ray – Stage 0
2. Bilateral hilar lymphadenopathy (BHL) alone – Stage I
3. BHL in conjunction with lung changes – Stage II
4. Lung changes alone – Stage III.

About 50% of patients with sarcoidosis present with BHL alone when the differential diagnosis (see Case 15) seldom gives rise to any difficulty. Indeed when BHL occurs in association with erythema nodosum the clinical picture is virtually pathognomonic of sarcoidosis. By contrast, pulmonary involvement in sarcoidosis, with or without signs of extrathoracic involvement, can mimic a wide variety of disease states and will often need to be considered in the differential diagnosis of infective (e.g. tuberculosis, histoplasmosis, atypical pneumonia) and neoplastic disorders, 'connective tissue' diseases and systemic vasculitides (see below). Compared to patients of Caucasian origin West Indians like Mr Benjamin – born abroad but resident in the UK – experience a far greater prevalence of the disease which is some six to seven times that of the indigenous population. They manifest erythema nodosum less often but they more commonly suffer from widespread disease and show a greater frequency of skin infiltrations, peripheral lymphadenopathy and eye changes compared with Caucasians.

In the absence of pulmonary fibrosis, the abnormal radiographic shadowing in sarcoidosis (corresponding to the granulomatous inflammatory infiltrate) usually conforms to one of three main patterns. The commonest appearance consists of widespread 'mottling' due to more or less evenly distributed micronodular shadows (less than 2 mm diameter) when miliary tuberculosis, extrinsic allergic alveolitis and pneumoconiosis enter the radiological differential diagnosis. In other cases the shadowing consists of larger (3–5 mm diameter), less well defined and more irregularly shaped and distributed nodules when the appearances more closely resemble those due to metastatic tumour infiltration (Figure A9.1). A third pattern is produced by large confluent areas of homogeneous shadowing which may be well or poorly defined ('cloudy shadowing'). Extensive shadowing may obscure the hilar regions and effectively mask hilar lymphadenopathy as in the case of Mr Benjamin (Figure A9.2), when the appearances may be attributed to infective consolidation, especially when febrile symptoms are also present.

Joint involvement in sarcoidosis most commonly takes the form of a febrile arthropathy, usually in the early stages of the disease when BHL is a common accompanying feature. This is characteristically a symmetrical polyarthritis which tends to be of limited

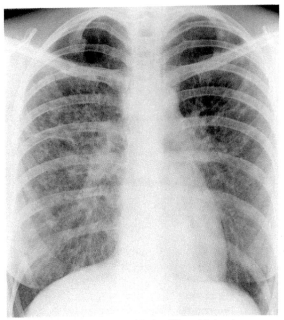

Figure A9.1 Pulmonary sarcoidosis: diffuse bilateral coarse nodular shadowing

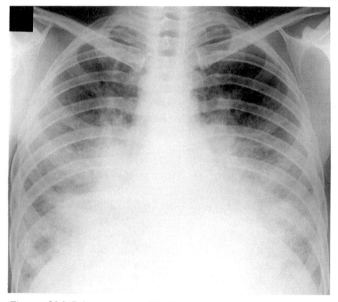

Figure A9.2 Pulmonary sarcoidosis: bilateral confluent mid and lower zone consolidation ('cloudy shadowing'), obscuring hilar shadows

duration, usually between two and three months. In some cases it may be more persistent or recurrent. The clinical picture is unlikely to be confused with rheumatoid disease except in those cases where erythema nodosum is absent and BHL inconspicuous. Pulmonary involvement in rheumatoid disease usually occurs relatively late and is almost invariably preceded by joint symptoms with an onset which tends to have been some years, rather than weeks or months, prior to the development of chest symptoms. Furthermore, the fibrosing alveolitis complicating rheumatoid disease is associated with progressive breathlessness, prominent respiratory signs (basal end-inspiratory lung crackles, finger clubbing), impaired lung function (restrictive ventilatory defect with reduced gas transfer) and a radiographic picture (bilateral reticulo-nodular shadowing most marked at the lung bases) which is distinct from that of sarcoidosis. By contrast, breathlessness is commonly trivial or absent despite the wide-spread radiographic changes that characterize the acute stage of sarcoidosis; clinical signs also tend to be minimal and crackles, in particular, are usually absent while significant disturbance of lung function is unusual. It must be remembered of course that a positive latex fixation test for rheumatoid factor is a not uncommon, non-specific manifestation of the hyperglobulinaemia that typifies sarcoidosis; high titres may be found especially in black subjects and in those with florid widespread sarcoidosis.

Bilateral pulmonary infiltrates, joint involvement and skin lesions also complicate the course of a variety of other connective tissue disorders (systemic sclerosis, systemic lupus erythematosus, dermatomyositis) where the clinical setting is unlikely to cause confusion with sarcoidosis.

A systemic vasculitis might also produce a similar picture. However, the description of Mr Benjamin's skin lesions is quite unlike the punched-out necrotic or purpuric lesions that are more characteristic of vasculitis. Lung involvement is uncommon in Henoch–Schönlein purpura, Behçet's disease and giant cell arteritis and most often complicates the vasculitis of polyarteritis (Churg–Strauss syndrome) and Wegener's granulomatosis. In the latter case the almost invariable presence of glomerulonephritis as well as symptoms (e.g. sinusitis, nasal obstruction and discharge) of upper as well as lower respiratory tract involvement serves to differentiate from sarcoidosis; the upper respiratory tract is commonly involved in sarcoidosis but associated symptomatology is unusual. Churg–Strauss syndrome may be recognized by virtue of its common association with atopic diseases, especially allergic rhinitis, eosinophilia and a history of asthma , frequently severe, which often precedes other evidence of systemic disease by months to several years.

Further reading

SCADDING J. G. and MITCHELL D. N. (1985) *Sarcoidosis.* Chapman and Hall, London.

Case 10

Answers

1. Alveolar cell carcinoma.
2. Lung biopsy (either transbronchial or percutaneous needle biopsy).
3. The outlook in cases of such advanced disease is very poor.

The term alveolar cell carcinoma is applied to a heterogeneous group of primary bronchial neoplasms which present similar gross and light microscopic appearances and which arise in the lung periphery. As currently defined the condition is not a single entity, referring as it does to a characteristic histological pattern (a peripheral tumour with growth of malignant cells along alveolar walls and an intact interstitial framework) without any precise histogenetic connotation. A variety of synonyms have been used, most commonly bronchiolo-alveolar cell carcinoma a term which emphasizes the peripheral location of the tumour and its uncertain histogenesis.

In most cases the tumours are morphologically identical to adenocarcinomas but electron microscopic observations suggest that, in some cases, the cell of origin may be the type II (granular) pneumocyte or the Clara cell. Some tumours show mixed morphology suggesting an origin from uncommitted bronchiolar stem cells. An identical histological pattern may be produced by extrathoracic tumours metastasizing to the lung, particularly gastrointestinal and pancreatic neoplasms. The diagnosis of primary alveolar cell carcinoma of the lung therefore presupposes the absence of a primary extrathoracic adenocarcinoma as determined either by a thorough clinical or postmortem examination.

In common with other lung adenocarcinomas the condition is less closely smoking-related than squamous and small cell anaplastic bronchial carcinomas and the sex ratio is approximately equal with only a slight predominance of males. Pre-existing lung disease, both focal (e.g. localized scarring secondary to tuberculosis, bronchiectasis, lung abscess, pulmonary infarction) and diffuse (e.g. rheumatoid lung, cryptogenic fibrosing alveolitis), is present in a high proportion of patients and may predispose to the development of the tumour. A viral aetiology has been suggested on the basis of clinical and histological similarities between human alveolar cell carcinoma and 'Jaagsiekte', an infectious disease of sheep, the latter having been linked to infection with viruses resembling RNA tumour viruses. The hypothesis is unproven and requires further study.

Alveolar cell carcinomas account for about 5% of all lung cancers. Patients characteristically present in the sixth or seventh decade. The clinical features (cough, dyspnoea, weight loss, chest pain) are similar to those of other lung cancers except that haemoptysis occurs less frequently and a higher proportion, up to 45%, are diagnosed at the stage of an asymptomatic peripheral opacity on a routine chest X-ray. Copious sputum production (bronchorrhoea) featured prominently in the present case and is often cited as a classical manifestation, but in fact it occurs only rarely and generally as a late manifestation.

The radiological features are variable. Early lesions give rise to a single peripheral opacity which is usually 1–10 cm in diameter and alveolar cell carcinoma must therefore be considered in the differential diagnosis of radiographic 'coin' lesions. A second type of appearance is produced by widely disseminated tumour deposits of variable size (ranging from miliary to 3–4 cm diameter), resulting in widespread nodular shadowing when miliary tuberculosis, sarcoidosis and secondary carcinoma will need to be considered in the wide differential diagnosis. A third pattern, that seen in the present case, relates to diffuse 'pneumonic' consolidation corresponding to the morbid anatomical appearance which resembles lobar pneumonia in the stage of grey hepatization. The absence of febrile symptoms, negative microbiological investigations and the persistence or progression of the radiographic shadowing should suggest the diagnosis of alveolar cell carcinoma. Occasionally the radiographic appearances mimic those of pulmonary oedema, pulmonary haemmorhage or alveolar proteinosis.

The diagnosis is usually made by lung biopsy. Because of the peripheral location of the tumour bronchoscopy is usually normal. Cytological investigations have given variable results. In general, examination of sputum, bronchial brushings and broncho-alveolar lavage fluid gives good results in patients with disseminated disease but is of little value in patients with a solitary nodule. Similarly, transbronchial biopsy gives a high diagnostic yield in patients with multinodular or diffuse disease but is less rewarding in the case of the solitary peripheral tumour for which percutaneous fine needle biopsy is the investigation of choice. However many such cases are diagnosed only at thoracotomy.

The outlook is generally favourable in patients presenting with localized disease and rather better than for other bronchogenic neoplasms, with a five year postoperative survival of around 50%. Unresectable disease carries a poor prognosis especially among elderly patients. Radiotherapy and chemotherapy are of no proven value and various measures (atropine, steroids, stellate ganglion block) aimed at controlling bronchorrhoea are generally found to be ineffective.

Further reading

EDWARDS, C. W. (1984) Alveolar carcinoma: a review. *Thorax*, **39**, 166.

Case 11

Answers

1. Primary bronchial carcinoma, arising at a peripheral location within the bronchial tree. (Following thoracotomy and lobectomy the tumour proved to be an adenocarcinoma).
2. The pattern of increased radioisotope uptake is in keeping with clinical findings suggesting hypertrophic pulmonary osteoarthropathy and must not be misinterpreted as being indicative of bony metastases.

Finger clubbing may occur in association with a wide variety of disease states but its most common cause is carcinoma of the bronchus where it is a feature in about 30% of new cases. It most commonly accompanies squamous cell tumours but may develop in association with any histological variety, although it is an unusual feature of small cell anaplastic lung cancer. Hypertrophic pulmonary osteoarthropathy (HPOA) is a closely related phenomenon which has as its two main features gross clubbing affecting the fingers and toes and periostitis with new bone formation characteristically affecting the long limb bones. HPOA too is most commonly associated with bronchial carcinoma but it may also occur with most of the potential causes of finger clubbing. As with simple finger clubbing, HPOA may complicate any histological cell type, but adenocarcinoma is implicated in about 25–30% of cases, a disproportionately high incidence. When gynaecomastia occurs in association with HPOA the tumour type is nearly always an adenocarcinoma. A variety of mechanisms has been suggested, but the pathogenesis of both clubbing and HPOA remains uncertain. Both disorders regress, often dramatically, following successful treatment of the primary tumour.

Apart from clubbing, which is occasionally absent, the characteristic clinical findings in HPOA consist of painful periarticular or joint swellings over the wrists, knees, ankles or elbows. These changes are often accompanied by joint effusions and abnormal sweating affecting the palms and soles. Joint swelling and tenderness may be associated with morning stiffness, mimicking rheumatoid arthritis, and a symptomatic response to non-steroidal anti-inflammatory drugs may appear to confirm this diagnosis. Any doubt is usually resolved by the distinctive radiographic appearances of HPOA; these are generally most readily observed in the distal shafts of the radius, ulna, tibia and fibula – 1–2 mm wide line shadows running parallel to the bone cortex (candlegrease appearance). Similar changes are often seen affecting the distal third of the metacarpal bones and the proximal and middle phalanges. The terminal phalanges usually show no radiographic abnormality even when finger clubbing is gross. Typically, the serum alkaline phosphatase is moderately elevated.

Confusion with rheumatoid disease is greatest in unusual cases where joint symptoms predominate and the radiographic changes of periostitis are inconspicuous, especially when clubbing is absent. In contrast to rheumatoid arthritis the synovial fluid in HPOA has been found to be 'non-inflammatory' with a low leucocyte count and few neutrophils, offering a further means of differentiation. The presence of rheumatoid factor in low titre is not unusual among elderly patients (present in about 10% of patients over 60 years) and is of no significance in Mrs MacKie's case except inasmuch that it could conceivably have been a source of diagnostic confusion. In practice a greater potential problem is confusion with bone metastases, a difficulty largely overcome by bone scanning. In HPOA high-quality radionuclide images will show pericortical deposition in contrast to the central increase in the concentration of the radioisotope that characterizes bony metastases.

Primary adenocarcinomas account for about 20% of malignant bronchial neoplasms. They are less closely smoking related than either squamous or small cell anaplastic tumours and, relative to these cell types, they are encountered more frequently among women. Adenocarcinoma is the predominant cell type in tumours complicating the course of diffuse interstitial pulmonary fibrosis (fibrosing alveolitis is associated with a tenfold increase in the incidence of bronchial carcinoma). Some so-called 'scar' adeno-carcinomas appear to develop at the site of pre-existing focal lung fibrosis which may also therefore predispose to this tumour type.

The vast majority of adenocarcinomas (80–90%) arise in the lung periphery and have no obvious relation to bronchi except by local invasion, compression or submucosal lymphatic permeation. They are relatively slowly growing tumours, but because of their peripheral origin they frequently reach a large size before causing symptoms and they often present, more commonly than is the case with other tumour types, as an incidental abnormality during routine radiological examination. As a corollary a preoperative diagnosis is established less frequently than with more central neoplasms: bronchoscopy and sputum cytology are usually negative, either transbronchial biopsy or percutaneous needle biopsy being more likely to provide a tissue diagnosis. Relatively more patients with an adenocarcinoma are judged to be operable after initial assessment and are found to have resectable disease at thoracotomy. Despite this, with the exception of alveolar cell carcinoma (see Case 10), the postoperative five year survival is poorer than for squamous carcinoma. This is due to the greater propensity among adenocarcinomas for haematogenous dissemination which, unsuspected at the time of surgery, results in a high rate of early (within the first two years of resection) postoperative deaths from metastatic disease.

Further reading

SMYTH, J. F. (1984) Editor. *The Management of Lung Cancer.* Edward Arnold, London.

Case 12

Answers

1. Pulmonary emphysema. Given the severity of the condition, its early onset in this patient and the lower zone predominance of the radiographic changes emphysema is almost certainly the result of α_1-antitrypsin deficiency.
2. Confirmation of this diagnosis rests on measurement of the serum level of α_1-antitrypsin (α_1-proteinase inhibitor or α_1-Pi). Very low levels (about 10–20% of normal) are characteristic of the most severely affected patients i.e. those homozygous for the Z phenotype (see below).
3. There is an autosomal recessive pattern of inheritance. The siblings of an index case (about one in four of whom will be affected) should be screened for the disorder. Their identification should be followed by vigorous counselling to avoid smoking and occupations associated with atmospheric pollution. Children who have one homozygous parent (phenotype PiZ) will inherit at least one 'Z' gene, i.e. they will all be heterozygotes. Genetic counselling should avoid pairing with another heterozygote with its attendant risk of producing homozygous alpha-1 antitrypsin deficient offspring.

Pulmonary emphysema is currently defined as a condition of the lung characterized by abnormal permanent enlargement of air spaces distal to the terminal bronchioles (compared with their size in normal lungs) with destruction of their walls, but without obvious fibrosis. It is strictly a condition that can only be diagnosed histologically. Clinical, radiographic and physiological changes give imprecise information in individual cases, but the combination of abnormalities can be sufficiently suggestive of emphysema to make a reasonably confident diagnosis during life and this is so in the case of Mr Gibson. (Recently, it has been claimed that accurate *in vivo* diagnosis of emphysema is possible by measuring the radioabsorbence of lung tissue using a method based upon the quantitative use of computed tomography).

The findings on clinical examination – signs of hyperinflation, wheeze and reduced breath sounds – are common to any cause of obstructive lung disease, including bronchial asthma. The same is true of a reduced FEV_1, a decreased FEV/FVC ratio and evidence of air trapping. The carbon monoxide diffusing capacity can help to discriminate to some extent in that total gas transfer (TL_{co}) is reduced in chronic obstructive bronchitis while the K_{co} is usually well preserved. In emphysema the characteristic finding is of reduction in both TL_{co} and K_{co}, the latter abnormality correlating

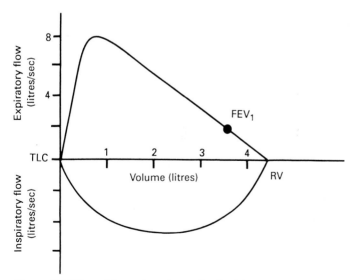

Figure A12.1 Normal flow volume-loop: triangle sitting on a semi-circle

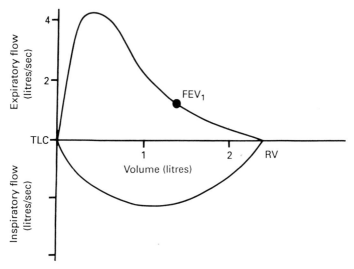

Figure A12.2 Flow-volume loop in volume-dependent airflow limitation: normal inspiratory limb, 'scooped out' expiratory limb

fairly well with the anatomical degree of emphysema. In bronchial asthma the effect on TL_{co} is variable, but the K_{co} is often increased.

The flow-volume relationship can also give a clue to the presence of emphysema. The normal relationship between flow and volume is depicted in Figure A12.1. Diffuse intrathoracic airway narrowing from any cause produces increased resistance to airflow and a reduction in maximum flow at all lung volumes, especially on expiration. The flow-volume loop may show a gradual 'scooping out' of the expiratory limb when the airways collapse progressively with expiration: volume-dependent airflow limitation (Figure A12.2). If the intrathoracic airways collapse immediately expiration begins, there is an abrupt fall from peak flow: pressure dependent airflow limitation (Figure A12.3). Emphysema is very likely to be present when, in the presence of a low K_{co}, the ratio of mid-inspiratory to mid-expiratory flow exceeds 10:1.

Of course the different types of obstructive lung disease are not mutually exclusive. They commonly coexist. The hallmark of asthma is its marked diurnal variability and reversibility in time or in response to treatment. The diagnosis is most readily apparent therefore not from a single set of lung function results, but from a

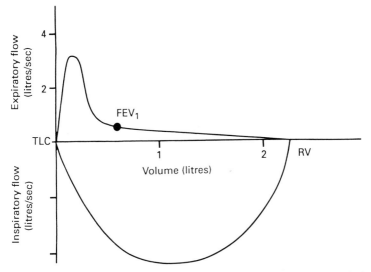

Figure A12.3 Flow-volume loop in severe pressure-dependent airflow limitation: abrupt early fall from peak flow; deep inspiratory limb

continuous domiciliary record of peak expiratory flow measurements. Even apparently persistent and progressive airways obstruction, a more characteristic course in chronic obstructive bronchitis or emphysema, may however prove to be reversible. A trial of oral corticosteroids (40 mg of prednisolone per day for two weeks) will identify a steroid responsive, 'asthmatic' component and can be justified in virtually all patients with airways obstruction whose symptoms are inadequately controlled with bronchodilator therapy. Even marked loss of gas transfer is not necessarily associated with a poor response to steroids.

The 'purest' cases of emphysema are seen in patients, like Mr Gibson, with α_1-antitrypsin deficiency. Among these patients smoking exerts a markedly synergistic effect in terms of its deleterious effect on lung function and it is usual therefore to see evidence of smoking related bronchial disease as well as purely emphysematous features. The normal phenotype (PiM) is conferred by inheritance of two 'M' protease inhibitor (Pi) genes. A variety of abnormal genes may code for α_1-antitrypsin: the PiZ phenotype results when an individual is homozygous for the abnormal recessive 'Z' gene. This is associated with very low serum levels of α_1-antitrypsin and affected individuals are at high risk of developing emphysema in middle age. There is also a greater than normal risk of hepatic cirrhosis and primary liver cancer in adult life, while about 10% of type 'Z' homozygotes develop evidence of hepatitis or cholestatic jaundice during the neonatal period. Heterozygotes (e.g. those with a PiMZ phenotype) show moderate reductions in serum antiprotease activity and increased susceptibility to emphysema would be expected. However population studies have failed to reveal an increase in symptomatic airways disease among heterozygotes. Nevertheless, the association of emphysema with severe antiprotease deficiency has led to the more general theory that emphysema in other individuals (independent of Pi phenotype) results from a subtle imbalance of proteolytic and antiproteolytic enzyme activity within the lung. Such an imbalance may, for example, be produced by cigarette smoking which not only inhibits the action of antiproteases but also promotes the attraction of enzyme-rich polymorphonuclear leucocytes and then stimulates the release of their potent proteolytic enzymes (Flenley, 1986).

Deficiency of α_1-antitrypsin has contributed greatly to our understanding of the pathogenesis of emphysema, but it is a rare cause of chronic respiratory disease. The prevalence of type 'Z' homozygotes among the newborn population has been estimated at 0.03%. Affected individuals suffer an early onset of respiratory symptoms, usually between the ages of 30 and 45. Apart from this earlier onset, the clinical and physiological features are similar to those in cases of emphysema in patients with normal levels of α_1-antitrypsin. The radiological findings, however, will sometimes suggest α_1-antitrypsin deficient emphysema when changes predominate in the lower zones. This contrasts with the more frequent involvement of the upper zones in emphysematous subjects with normal levels of α_1-antitrypsin.

Reference and further reading

FLENLEY, D. C. (1986) Pathogenesis of pulmonary emphysema. *The Quarterly Journal of Medicine*, **61**, 901.

TOBIN, M. J., COOK, P. J. L. and HUTCHISON, D. C. S. (1983) α_1-antitrypsin deficiency: the clinical and physiological features of pulmonary emphysema in subjects homozygous for Pi type Z. A survey by the British Thoracic Association. *British Journal of Diseases of the Chest*, **77**, 14.

Case 13

Answers

1. Mrs Mayhew's clinical deterioration is probably the result of secondary infection by *Aspergillus fumigatus*.
2. An aspergilloma might be more readily identifiable in tomographic views of the lung apices. Positive serum precipitins to *Aspergillus fumigatus* confirms fungal colonization.

The symptom complex – productive cough, haemoptysis and weight loss – engenders a wide differential diagnosis when the affected patient is a smoker with a previous history of pulmonary tuberculosis. Mrs Mayhew's fear of recurrent tuberculosis must be considered along with the possibility of bronchial carcinoma and secondary infection due either to opportunistic organisms or as a complication of post-tuberculous bronchiectasis.

Cavitation in cases of active postprimary pulmonary tuberculosis is nearly always associated with smear positive disease (tubercle bacilli seen on microscopy of sputum) and repeatedly negative direct examination of purulent sputum is strongly against the diagnosis of recurrent disease. Furthermore, Mrs Mayhew had been treated for tuberculosis some years before. Whilst late relapses (two years or more after the cessation of antituberculous chemotherapy) do occur, they are relatively rare, by far the majority of treatment failures being apparent within two years of stopping therapy. Relapse is also unlikely when treatment has included the strong bactericidal combination of rifampicin and isoniazid, particularly when it is known to have been for an adequate duration and associated with good compliance. Mrs Mayhew's fear would appear ill-founded.

Bronchiectasis is an almost invariable complication of postprimary tuberculosis. However, it is unusual for this to result in clinical symptoms because it is the upper lobes, which are well drained by gravity, that are most often affected. Secondary infection is far more likely to arise in a patient in whom treatment has been otherwise successful but has resulted in a large residual cavity. About 70–80% of tuberculous cavities close under the influence of effective chemotherapy and those that persist are usually asymptomatic. In a proportion of cases secondary bacterial infection or fungal colonization supervenes. In Mrs Mayhew's case the identification in the sputum of *Aspergillus fumigatus*, in the absence of any other pathogens, strongly suggests an aspergillo-ma. The diagnosis was confirmed by X-ray tomography of the right apex showing multiple mycetomas and by the presence of strongly positive serum precipitins against *Aspergillus fumigatus*. A peripheral cavitating bronchial carcinoma arising in tuberculous scar tissue (usually an adenocarcinoma: so-called 'scar cancer') or arising, coincidentally, in association with an aspergilloma cannot be definitively excluded on the basis of the case history. Negative cytological investigations render neoplasm less likely whilst the distinctive radiographic appearances of mycetoma serve to exclude any residual doubt.

The vast majority of mycetomas are encountered in the apical segments of the upper lobes, a reflection of the fact that most arise as a late complication of tuberculous cavitation. In one large survey of patients with healed tuberculosis, aspergillomas developed in 15% of residual cavities. The highest incidence was found in cavities of 7–11 years' duration. Other predisposing causes include sarcoidosis, ankylosing spondylitis, allergic bronchopulmonary aspergillosis, postradiation fibrosis, lung abscess, bronchiectasis and bullous emphysema. In about 20% of cases aspergillomas are multiple.

Serum precipitins to *Aspergillus fumigatus* are almost invariable and the strength of the precipitation reaction can be of diagnostic value in relation to the clinical type of infection. Aspergillomas characteristically give rise to multiple, easily identifiable precipitin lines in the immunoprecipitation reaction. By contrast, in allergic bronchopulmonary aspergillosis, precipitin lines are fewer in number and less well defined; precipitins are usually absent in immunocompromised patients with invasive aspergillosis.

Immediate skin prick tests are positive in about 70% of patients with mycetoma. Asthmatic features are common and a small proportion of patients satisfy the criteria for allergic bronchopul-monary aspergillosis. Chronic productive cough and dyspnoea are common features and frequently reflect the underlying lung disease or secondary bacterial infection. Haemoptysis which may be life threatening occurs at some stage in the majority of patients. Systemic features of weight loss, fever and malaise are found in a small proportion of cases, usually those with large mycetomas. Rarely, an invasive aspergillus infection supervenes, a condition most commonly associated with severely immunocompromized patients.

The treatment of aspergillomas is unsatisfactory. Surgical resection is associated with an operative mortality of about 7% and major complications (haemorrhage, bronchopleural fistula, empyema) in a similar proportion of patients. The approach should be reserved for patients with severe haemoptysis and good pulmonary reserve. The majority of patients are unfit for surgery because of compromised lung function. Recurrent severe haemoptysis can sometimes be successfully treated among such patients by means of bronchial arterial embolization. Intracavitary instillation of antifungal drugs has given variable results, while systemic antifungal therapy is without benefit except in the rare cases of associated invasive aspergillosis.

Further reading

A REPORT FROM THE RESEARCH COMMITTEE OF THE BRITISH THORACIC AND TUBERCULOSIS ASSOCIATION (1970). Aspergilloma and residual tuberculous cavities – the results of a resurvey. *Tubercle*, **51,** 227.

JEWKES, J., KAY, P. H., PANETH, M. and CITRON, K. (1983) Pulmonary aspergilloma: an analysis of prognosis in relation to haemoptysis and survey of treatment. *Thorax*, **38,** 572.

RAFFERTY, P., BIGGS, P. A., CROMPTON, G. K. and GRANT, I. W. B. (1983) What happens to patients with pulmonary aspergilloma? Analysis of 23 cases. *Thorax*, **38,** 579.

Case 14

Answers

1. A chylous effusion.
2. Malignant lymphoma.

Pleural effusions may be rendered opaque by the presence of blood or by the accumulation of leucocytes (empyema), fat droplets (chylous effusion) or cholesterol crystals (pseudochylous effusion). Pus bears only a superficial resemblance to the characteristic white, 'milky' appearance of chylous fluid and the clinical setting will usually render differentiation from an empyema clear cut. Any doubt will be resolved by the use of fat stains which are taken up by chylous fluid, by bench centrifugation (chylous effusions will have a clear supernatant), or by microscopy.

Pseudochylous effusions occur as a complication of chronic pleural collections (e.g. secondary to tuberculosis, rheumatoid disease, nephrotic syndrome, carcinoma), when the accumulation of cholesterol crystals and other debris gives rise to a turbid, opalescent fluid which may appear to shimmer when inspected by transmitted light. They may also appear 'milky' when they are more readily confused with chylous fluid. The use of fat stains and microscopic identification of fat globules in chylous effusions serve to differentiate.

A chylous effusion (chylothorax) may result from any condition causing disruption of the thoracic duct. The latter extends from its origin in the abdomen (the cisterna chyli, which lies in front of the upper two lumbar vertebrae), through the aortic opening of the diaphragm and the posterior mediastinum to the root of the neck where, most commonly, it enters the venous system at the junction of the left internal jugular and subclavian veins. Although a comparatively rare condition, it has become more common in recent years owing to the increasing frequency of thoracic surgery. The majority of chylous effusions, about half, are secondary to malignant disease. Approximately 25% are traumatic in origin and the remainder are of varied aetiology (Table A14.1).

Traumatic chylous effusions are usually the result of intrathoracic surgery particularly surgery in close proximity to the left subclavian artery. By comparison, chylothorax complicates various forms of accidental trauma only very rarely. Malignant chylous effusions are usually the result of a lymphoma with tumour infiltration of the thoracic duct or left subclavian vein. Less commonly, metastatic deposits from a wide range of primary sites, especially stomach, may be responsible. In the case described, this diagnosis was in fact suspected given the patient's strong family history of stomach cancer, but a negative barium meal examination made this diagnosis highly unlikely. A diagnosis of non-Hodgkin's lymphoma was established from biopsies obtained during diagnostic thoracotomy.

Characteristically, chylous effusions rapidly recur following aspiration and, because the volume of chyle produced each day may be as great as 2.5 litres, repeated aspiration results in clinical deterioration with fat, electrolyte and water depletion, hypo-proteinaemia and lymphopenia. Conservative treatment, where nutritional support (intravenous feeding) and drainage of the effusion is followed by the promotion of a pleurodesis (e.g. using talc or tetracycline), can be successful in preventing further accumulation of chyle. When this approach fails surgical ligation of

Table A14.1 Causes of chylous pleural effusion (chylothorax)

Malignant (50%)
Lymphoma
Metastatic carcinoma

Traumatic (25%)
Surgical trauma, e.g.
    intrathoracic operations
    cervical lymph node dissections
Non-surgical trauma, e.g.
    penetrating injuries
    blunt chest/abdominal injuries
    birth injury during traumatic delivery

Infectious
Tuberculous mediastinal lymphadenitis
Filariasis

Congenital (very rare)
Multiple thoracic duct fistulae

Miscellaneous
Thoracic aortic aneurysm
Left subclavian vein thrombosis
Benign lymphangioma of the thoracic duct
Lymphangioleiomyomatosis

the thoracic duct offers safe and effective treatment and should be considered early. In Mr Daniels' case it proved impossible to approach the thoracic duct at thoracotomy because of the extent of his tumour. Fortunately, treatment with chemotherapy and subsequently mediastinal irradiation led to closure of the fistula and there was no subsequent recurrence of his chylothorax.

Further reading

BESSONE L. N., FERGUSON T. B. and BURFORD T. H. (1971) Chylothorax. *The Annals of Thoracic Surgery*, **12**, 527.
ROBINSON C. L. N. (1985) The Management of chylothorax. *The Annals of Thoracic Surgery*, **39**, 90.

Case 15

Answers

1. There is bilateral hilar and right sided paratracheal lymphadenopathy.
2. (a) Sarcoidosis.
   (b) Malignant lymphoma.
3. Cervical lymph node biopsy.

Table A15.1 lists the main causes of intrathoracic lymphadenopathy. Uncommon drug related causes (e.g. para-aminosalicylic acid, phenylbutazone, phenytoin) and lymphadenopathy associated with the pneumoconioses, silicosis and berylliosis, will be suggested by a patient's drug and occupational history, respectively. Acute (primary) and chronic progressive forms of both histoplasmosis and coccidioidomycosis enter the differential diagnosis of hilar and mediastinal lymphadenopathy in endemic regions (e.g. United States). In the UK pulmonary tuberculosis and, especially among children or young adults, whooping cough and infectious mononucleosis are the only commonly encountered infective causes. In the present case the absence of cough or febrile symptoms and the rather prolonged clinical course would tend to exclude these two latter possibilities. This would also be an unusual presentation of tuberculosis in an adult Caucasian where tuberculous cervical lymphadenitis is most frequently encountered in the absence of any signs of active pulmonary tuberculosis. This contrasts with clinical presentations of tuberculosis among patients of Asian extraction where there may be pronounced and extensive lymphadenopathy complicating pulmonary disease. In Mrs Terry's case the negative tuberculin reaction provides further evidence against a diagnosis of tuberculosis.

In clinical practice in the UK adult patients presenting with a combination of cervical and intrathoracic lymphadenopathy are likely to be suffering from either sarcoidosis, malignant lymphoma or 'carcinomatosis'. Patients with sarcoidosis generally appear in good health and, like Mrs Terry, commonly have no, or only trivial, systemic symptoms. Patients with malignant disease on the other hand are usually systemically unwell and, in the case of metastatic tumours, there are usually symptoms or signs pointing to the underlying primary.

Table A15.1   Causes of intrathoracic lymphadenopathy

Sarcoidosis
Pulmonary tuberculosis
Certain bacterial, viral and fungal infections, e.g.
    whooping cough, infectious mononucleosis,
    histoplasmosis, coccidioidomycosis
Malignant lymphoma and leukaemia
Metastatic neoplasms
Silicosis
Berylliosis
Drug idiosyncrasy

The specific radiological features may be of diagnostic value when, in the case of metastatic disease, hilar adenopathy is associated with the typical radiographic appearances of lymphangitis carcinomatosa (see Answer 1). Sarcoidosis characteristically produces bilateral, symmetrical hilar lymph node enlargement. Lymphadenopathy is usually moderate and seldom massive. Associated paratracheal lymphadenopathy, usually right-sided, is present in excess of 50% of cases but tends to be modest and only rarely overshadows the hilar component. In malignant lymphomas, as in sarcoidosis, lymphadenopathy is usually bilateral, but is often asymmetrical; hilar nodes are seldom involved in isolation and they are often overshadowed by more frequent and prominent involvement of paratracheal and tracheobronchial lymph nodes.

Erythema nodosum and/or febrile arthropathy commonly accompany the acute stages of bilateral hilar lymphadenopathy (BHL) in sarcoidosis, especially in women, when the clinical picture is virtually pathognomonic and tissue biopsy is generally held to be superfluous provided that there are no discordant features. Depression of delayed hypersensitivity responses to 'recall' antigens is characteristic of sarcoidosis but is also a feature of lymphoproliferative disorders. Mrs Terry's tuberculin anergy, although it is consistent with sarcoidosis (and renders tuberculosis highly improbable), it does not differentiate from malignant lymphoma. Splenomegaly too is a feature of both disorders. In Mrs Terry's case therefore the clinical features alone are not diagnostic and, in these circumstances, confirmatory investigations are mandatory.

Scadding and Mitchell (1985) have pointed out that, for the clinician, 'the diagnosis of sarcoidosis is a statement of belief or knowledge that non-caseating epitheloid cell tubercles or their hyalinized remnants are present in a number of affected organs or tissues.' The diagnosis will be supported by a wide variety of clinical, radiological, biochemical (raised serum levels of angiotensin-converting enzyme and lysozyme, hyperglobulin-aemia, hyercalcaemia, hypercalcuria) and immunological findings (e.g. tuberculin anergy, positive Kveim test, a high proportion of activated T-lymphocytes in broncho-alveolar lavage fluid), but the diagnosis is rendered most secure if a compatible clinical picture is corroborated by histological evidence of 'sarcoid' granulomatosis in at least one affected organ.

In general terms, the need for biopsy confirmation depends upon the degree of confidence with which the clinical diagnosis is made. Atypical clinical presentations may require that several sites of disease are biopsied for a confident diagnosis. Most often biopsy of a single site of disease involvement will suffice. Enlarged superficial lymph nodes and skin lesions commonly present readily accessible and convenient sources of biopsy material. In the presence of pulmonary infiltration transbronchial lung biopsy via the flexible bronchoscope is relatively non-invasive and gives a high diagnostic yield. It is characteristic of the early stages of sarcoidosis, however, that granulomas are widespread and 'random' biopsies of apparently unaffected tissue (e.g. nasal and bronchial mucosa, liver, skeletal muscle, salivary glands) will often show characteristic histological changes.

Reference

SCADDING J. G. and MITCHELL D. N. (1985) Sarcoidosis. Chapman and Hall, London.

Case 16

Answers

1. Malignant pleural mesothelioma.
2. Treatment should be symptomatic with an emphasis upon adequate control of pain and relief of breathlessness.
3. Malignant mesothelioma became a prescribed industrial disease in 1966. The patient or his dependents are eligible for compensation should the diagnosis be agreed by the Pneumoconiosis Medical Panel (Medical Boarding Centre) to which suspected cases should be referred for certification.

Malignant mesotheliomas are rare tumours with an estimated annual incidence of 1 per million population per year. They arise from the mesothelial lining of serosal cavities–pleura, peritoneum, pericardium and the tunica vaginalis of the testes. There is a close association with asbestos exposure, most tumours developing after a prolonged latent period averaging about 40 years after first exposure. The last two decades has seen a real increase in the incidence of mesotheliomas owing to the increasingly widespread use of asbestos in industry, especially during the 1930s and 1940s, when shipbuilding and ship-repairing yards were an important source of exposure.

Males predominate in all series (sex ratio of between 2:1 and 5:1) owing to the fact that they have been more frequently employed in the use of asbestos. However, women who were engaged in the wartime manufacture of gas-masks have shown a particularly high incidence of the disease. Non-occupational asbestos exposure (e.g. domestic exposure or 'neighbourhood' exposure among individuals living in the immediate vicinity of, for example, an asbestos factory) has been implicated in a small percentage of cases. The degree of exposure is therefore much less than that required to cause asbestosis.

The majority of tumours arise in the pleura, the ratio of pleural to peritoneal mesotheliomas being about 5:1. The remaining sites of origin are much less common. Pleural tumours involve both visceral and parietal pleura. Characteristically, the posterior and basal surfaces of the pleura, especially the diaphragmatic pleura, are the most prominent sites of tumour involvement. With progressive disease tumour extends along interlobar fissures, encasing and compressing the underlying lung. Histologically, mesotheliomas present a variable pattern and four distinct types can be recognized: tubo-papillary, sarcomatous, undifferentiated and mixed. Pathological diagnosis is often difficult on small samples obtained using pleural biopsy needles. This is especially so in the case of tubo-papillary tumours, the most common variety, where the histological pattern closely resembles that due to metastatic adenocarcinoma.

Typically the patient presents with an insidious onset, over weeks or months, of either non-pleuritic chest pain or breathlessness. Cough, haemoptysis and weight loss occur less often and finger clubbing occurs in fewer than 10% of cases. The patient often appears well and the clinical diagnosis frequently goes unsuspected for many months. An acute presentation with severe chest pain or dyspnoea is seen in about 5% of cases.

The usual finding on physical examination is of a large unilateral pleural effusion. The clinical course is marked by increasing chest pain and breathlessness as well as other features due to direct tumour growth (Horner's syndrome, brachial plexus involvement, pericardial and mediastinal invasion). Distant metastases are common at autopsy but are seldom clinically apparent. Tumour growth along needle tracks (e.g. following pleural aspiration or pleural biopsy) may result in painful chest wall masses and is often regarded as a characteristic feature. However, this complication was seen in only 11% of one large series of 327 patients (Elmes and Simpson, 1976) and its anticipation does not contraindicate either diagnostic pleural biopsy or therapeutic pleural aspiration.

Diagnostic success rests upon a high index of suspicion. Because of the prolonged latency of mesothelioma careful enquiry is often necessary to elicit a history of exposure to asbestos which is often both remote and of relatively short duration. The radiographic appearances (Figure A16.1), as described here, are typical and lend support to the diagnosis. This is especially the case when there are asbestos-related pleural or pulmonary changes (hyaline or calcified pleural plaques, pleural thickening

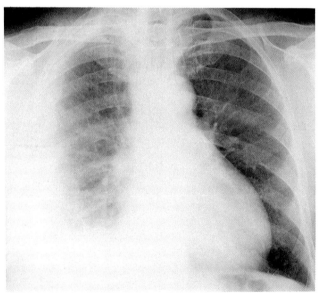

Figure A16.1 Pleural mesothelioma: extensive lobulated right sided pleural thickening

or changes due to asbestosis) in the contralateral hemithorax, which applies to about one-third of mesotheliomas. The radiographic appearances are not pathognomonic however. Many tumours can metastasize to the pleura and the definitive diagnosis of mesothelioma must obviously depend upon histological material.

Rarely, a patient will present with early, apparently localized disease when surgical cure may be possible by radical pleuro-pneumonectomy. For the vast majority of patients who present with advanced disease treatment is essentially palliative. Pain control requires adequate analgesic therapy. Pleural aspiration may afford symptomatic relief from breathlessness in the earlier stages of the disease; tumour growth progressively obliterates the pleural cavity and pleural fluid tends to absorb spontaneously so that both the need for and benefit from pleural aspiration diminishes as the disease advances. Neither radiotherapy nor chemotherapy are of any established value. The outlook is poor, patients surviving a median duration of about 12 months from the onset of symptoms.

Reference and further reading

ELMES, P. C. and SIMPSON, M. (1976) The clinical aspects of mesothelioma. *Quarterly Journal of Medicine*, **45**, 427.

LAW, M. R., GREGOR, A. HODSON, M. E. *et al.*, (1984) Malignant mesothelioma of the pleura; a study of 52 treated and 64 untreated patients. *Thorax*, **39**, 255.

Case 17

Answers

1. Right apical bronchial carcinoma (Pancoast or superior sulcus tumour).
2. (a) Pain due to brachial plexus involvement.
   (b) Right Horner's syndrome (the full syndrome consists of ptosis, miosis, enopthalmos and ipsilateral anhidrosis).
   (c) Spinal cord compression due to either metastatic disease or to direct tumour growth.

Henry Pancoast, an American radiologist, is credited with the first detailed description of the clinical syndrome which now bears his name. Pancoast believed that a specific tumour type was responsible. It is now understood that the syndrome is not a pathological entity but can be caused by a variety of expanding lesions, both benign and malignant, arising in the thoracic inlet. The superior pulmonary sulcus refers to the apex of the upper lobe and to the groove made by the subclavian artery in the cupola of the pleura. By virtue of its complex local anatomy even quite small lesions at this site may involve the lower trunks of the brachial plexus (with resulting pain and parasthesiae), the cervical sympathetic chain and stellate ganglion (with ipsilateral Horner's syndrome), and the roots of the eighth cervical and first and second thoracic nerves with possible local extension into adjacent ribs and vertebrae. Bronchial carcinoma is by far the commonest cause of the syndrome and about 2–4% of lung tumours, mostly squamous neoplasms, are thus complicated. Other recognized malignant causes include pleural mesothelioma, Hodgkin's disease and myelomatosis. Benign causes (e.g. pulmonary tuberculosis, hydatid disease, osteomyelitis/abscess of an adjacent rib or vertebral body) are rare but must not be overlooked.

The usual presentation is with pain which is often severe and apparent for some months prior to the onset of other features. Typically pain is felt initially in the shoulder and later extends to the elbow along the inside of the arm and subsequently along the ulnar aspect of the forearm to the fourth and fifth digits. Ultimately weakness and wasting may be noted affecting the intrinsic muscles of the hand. Anterior praecordial pain is present in some patients and with left-sided tumours, when there is radiation of pain to the left arm, there is the potential for confusion with myocardial ischaemia. The persistent nature of the pain and its lack of relation to exertion help to differentiate. More commonly patients are treated for cervical osteoarthritis, sometimes for months, before the correct diagnosis is made. In the present case, in spite of her previous tuberculous history, apical pulmonary tuberculosis is highly unlikely in a tuberculin negative subject with negative bacteriology. Occasionally plombage, used in the treatment of previous apical pulmonary tuberculosis, will mimic the radiographic appearance of a Pancoast tumour.

Mrs Carlyle's clinical presentation is therefore typical of most with symptoms and signs of local tumour invasion, very often occurring well in advance of any evidence of metastatic disease. In this case the patient's paraplegia, due to epidural spinal cord compression, was also the result of direct spread, with extension of tumour through the intervertebral foramina. Paraplegia complicates about 5% of all Pancoast neoplasms. Because of the peripheral location of these tumours, sputum cytology and brochoscopy are usually negative. A tissue diagnosis is most readily established by percutaneous needle biopsy.

Radiographically the apical abnormality is often small in relation to the severity of symptoms. It is frequently difficult to define and may not be demonstrable at all from plain radiographs. CT or conventional tomography may be of value. The typical appearance is that of an homogeneous mass density with an irregular lower margin. A well penetrated radiograph will often show destructive changes affecting the posterior aspects of one or more of the upper ribs, usually the first, second and third. Destructive changes affecting the articular and transverse processes and sometimes the bodies of one or more adjacent vertebrae are features of more advanced disease.

Historically, bronchial carcinomas arising in the superior sulcus have always been associated with a poor prognosis. Pancoast himself believed these tumours to be uniformly fatal, with no benefit associated with either surgery or radiotherapy. However, in the absence of regional lymph node and distant metastases, prolonged survival may in fact follow radical en-bloc resection. The best results are achieved when resection is combined with moderate doses of preoperative radiotherapy (30–40 Gy) which significantly improves the resectability rate. This aggressive approach is justifiable in a highly selected group of patients in whom staging procedures confirm the localized nature of the disease. For unresectable tumours – the majority of cases – and those with nodal or metastatic disease radical surgery is of no benefit and in these cases modern radiotherapy techniques offer good palliation.

Further reading

HOWARD, G. C. W. and BLEEHAN, N. M. (1983) Pancoast's syndrome. *British Journal of Hospital Medicine,* **29,** 496.

Case 18

Answers

1. Intrathoracic goitre.
2. The Empey Index is calculated by dividing the FEV_1 (in ml) by the PEFR (in l/min). This ratio is usually less than 10 in normal subjects and in patients with obstructive lung disease due to narrowing affecting intrapulmonary airways (asthma, chronic obstructive bronchitis and emphysema). A value greater than 10 suggests upper airway obstruction.

Localized narrowing affecting the upper (central) airway is seen much less frequently than *diffuse* intrathoracic airways obstruction. Clinical recognition of the problem is not always straightforward and delayed diagnosis is not uncommon with symptoms and signs of upper airway obstruction often misinterpreted as being the result of bronchial asthma or chronic bronchitis. Diagnostic difficulty is greatest if the two conditions (localized upper airway narrowing and diffuse intrathoracic airflow obstruction) co-exist when the localized lesion is particularly likely to go unrecognized. Accurate diagnosis is essential as there are important therapeutic implications. Surgical cure is the rule for 'benign' causes and treatment for localized malignant lesions in the upper airway is often associated with prolonged survival.

Stridor is the cardinal clinical feature of localized upper airway obstruction. Often, however, there is no abnormality during normal breathing or, as in the present case, there may be evidence of only noisy breath sounds (due to turbulent airflow). Stridor will often become apparent after exercise or during hyperventilation through the open mouth when, using the stethoscope, a fixed monophonic (single pitched) wheeze is audible over the trachea; becoming fainter when auscultating over the lungs. The intensity of the wheeze is maximal during inspiration (as with laryngeal obstruction) when the extrathoracic portion of the trachea – between the larynx and the thoracic inlet – is narrowed. The converse applies (i.e. wheeze more marked during expiration) to conditions causing narrowing of the intrathoracic portion of the trachea, distal to the thoracic inlet, when there is perhaps the greatest potential for misdiagnosing diffuse airways disease.

Flow-volume curves (see Answer 12) will nearly always show

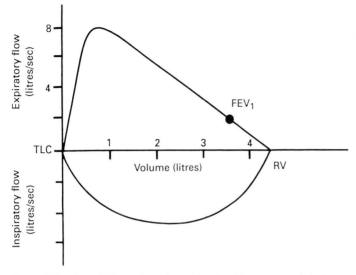

Figure A18.1 Normal Flow-volume loop: triangle sitting on a semi-circle

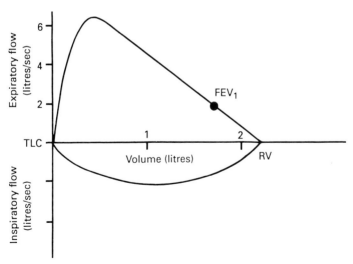

Figure A18.2 Flow-volume loop in 'variable' upper (extrathoracic) airway obstruction

distinctive changes and they offer valuable confirmatory evidence of central airway obstruction. The appearance of the curves is dependent upon the site and severity of the obstruction and also upon whether the lesion is fixed (when the airway is rigid and its walls immobile) or variable (with a mobile airway wall). The normal flow–volume relationship is depicted in Figure A18.1. Extrathoracic airway obstruction produces a curve similar to that in Figure A18.2 when the airway is mobile, e.g. bilateral vocal cord palsy. Maximum inspiratory flow is more limited than maximum expiratory flow (the converse applies in cases of diffuse intrathoracic obstruction – compare Figures A12.2 and A12.3). This is because during a forced inspiration the pressure in the extrathoracic airway falls below atmospheric which will favour collapse of the mobile walls of the partially obstructed airway. During forced expiration the intrathoracic pressure, and therefore the airway pressure, exceeds atmospheric which favours airway patency and, as a consequence, the expiratory limb appears normal.

A fixed extrathoracic airway obstruction (e.g. secondary to a fibrous stricture or tracheal tumour), when the walls of the airway are no longer mobile, results in limitation of both inspiratory and expiratory flows (Figure A18.3). Typically, the maximum flows that are most impaired are those that are most dependent upon effort. Inspiratory flow rates are reduced throughout the vital capacity,

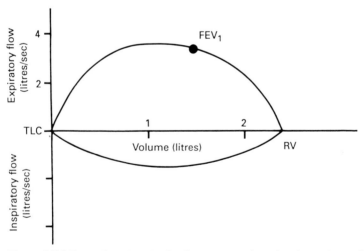

Figure A18.3 Flow-volume loop in 'fixed' upper (extrathoracic) airway obstruction

whereas the reduction in expiratory flow rates is most marked at higher lung volumes. This produces a blunted peak expiratory flow rate but a normal contour to the latter part of the expiratory limb (i.e. at low lung volumes) when flow is less effort dependent. The appearance is similar to that produced by an overall reduction in driving pressure due, for example, to respiratory muscle weakness when the clinical picture will serve to differentiate. A similar curve could also be produced if poor patient cooperation results in inadequate effort but, in this case, repeated measurements will tend to give inconsistent results.

Thus, simple inspection of the flow-volume curves can be highly instructive. Where this facility is not available other spirometric measurements will frequently offer clues to the presence of upper airway obstruction. The 'Empey' index, which requires knowledge of only the PEF and FEV_1, may provide one such clue. In upper airway obstruction the PEF is often unexpectedly low in relation to the FEV_1; this is because the latter effectively integrates maximum expiratory flows over both the effort-dependent and effort-independent portions of the flow-volume curve and it tends to be relatively insensitive to changes in central airway calibre. By contrast the PEF, which is completely effort-dependent, is characteristically reduced to a much greater extent.

Whenever localized upper airway obstruction is suspected a full assessment will require not only pulmonary function testing, but also careful endoscopic and radiological evaluation (including tomography of the trachea and larger bronchi) in order to define more precisely the site and severity of the lesion and to provide information concerning its likely aetiology. Table A18.1 lists the

Table A18.1   Causes of localized upper airway obstruction

Extrinsic compression due to:
Enlarged (malignant) lymph nodes
Mediastinal tumours, e.g. thymoma
Intrathoracic goitre
Vascular aneurysms

Intrinsic abnormalities
Primary tumours of the central airway, e.g. bronchial and tracheal carcinoma, cylindroma
Post-traumatic stricture, e.g. following intubation/tracheostomy
Granulomatous disorders: sarcoidosis, tuberculosis, Wegener's granulomatosis
Amyloidosis
Congenital atresia

main causes encountered in clinical practice, the commonest being primary tumours involving the central airway and extrinsic compression secondary to 'malignant' lymphadenopathy or other mediastinal tumours.

In Mrs Sands' case the plain radiograph (Figure A18.4) was sufficient to suggest the diagnosis of intrathoracic goitre. This typically produces a well defined homogeneous shadow occupying a high position in the superior mediastinum. Often, as in this case, the mass is asymmetrical and typically projects more to the right than the left. Marked asymmetry may cause confusion with vascular lesions; computed tomography with enhancement or angiography will differentiate. In addition, radioisotope uptake in the superior mediastinum will sometimes enable a confident diagnosis of intrathoracic goitre.

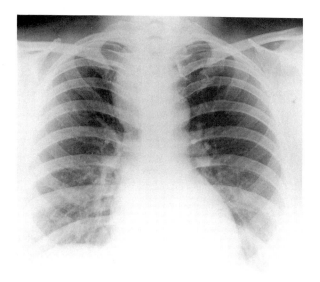

Figure A18.4 Intrathoracic goitre: well defined homogeneous mass with a smooth convex lateral margin projecting to the right in the superior mediastinum

Case 19

Answers

1. Primary bronchial carcinoma, probably of squamous cell type.
2. Treatment will be palliative and should be directed primarily, at least initially, toward the correction of hypercalcaemia. Subsequently, local radiotherapy may or may not be appropriate depending upon the presence or absence of tumour-related respiratory symptoms. It is doubtful whether chemotherapy would ever be appropriate for an inoperable squamous cell carcinoma in a man of this age.

Confusion, weight loss and recent impairment of mobility (the patient having 'gone off his feet') are common and highly non-specific indicators of disease among elderly patients, engendering a wide diagnostic spectrum which includes both physical and psychiatric disorders. When, as is so often the case, a reliable history is not possible careful physical examination and the results of simple investigations frequently prove to be most rewarding.

The pattern of haematological and biochemical abnormalities is a common one in myelomatosis, a diagnosis which could certainly account for the clinical presentation with confusion secondary to either hypercalcaemia or hyperviscosity. A raised serum alkaline phosphatase is unusual, however, except in the presence of healing fractures. The absence of proteinuria, the normal appearance of the ribs – a particularly common site for bone lesions in myelomatosis – and the normal bone scan all argue against this diagnosis. Nor would myelomatosis readily account for the patient's hoarse voice or for the radiographic abnormality of the left hilum which, in an elderly, heavy cigarette smoker (nicotine-stained fingers), strongly suggests recurrent laryngeal nerve palsy due to a central bronchial neoplasm.

The plain chest X-ray is an important diagnostic tool in bronchial carcinoma and is nearly always abnormal at the time of presentation. The commonest abnormality consists of unilateral hilar enlargement with or without associated distal collapse or consolidation. Gross hilar abnormalities are easy to interpret but subtle changes, which are readily reproduced by faulty radiographic technique (e.g. patient rotation) or in the presence of scoliosis, may also be significant. In properly performed and adequately penetrated X-rays a difference in the radiodensity of the two hilar shadows, slight loss of sharpness of a hilar outline or loss of the normal concave lateral aspect may be early evidence of disease. Radiographic interpretation of the lung hilum is largely a subjective exercise and is prone to observer error. Hilar tomography may help in the evaluation but in general, if there is clinical suspicion, the wisest course is to proceed to bronchoscopy.

A few radiographic pitfalls are worthy of note. A tumour arising in the apical segment of a lower lobe will be projected over the lung hilum in an anterior view film and thus simulate a hilar mass; a lateral view radiograph will differentiate. In a small proportion of cases the postero-anterior (PA) chest film appears normal. A standard X-ray will usually fail to resolve tumours less than 1 cm in diameter. Much lung tissue is also 'hidden' on a PA film being obscured by the heart or diaphragm and if the diagnosis is suspected a lateral view radiograph is mandatory. Small peripheral tumours may be obscured by a rib. Tumours at the carina or within a main bronchus are obscured by the central mediastinal shadow and may exceed 2 cm in diameter before becoming radiologically visible.

A normal radioisotope bone scan suggests, but does not exclude, the absence of skeletal spread of tumour and increases the likelihood that hypercalaemia is a non-metastatic phenomenon related to ectopic tumour production of humoral mediators. A variety of ectopic products may be implicated: parathyroid hormone, parathyroid hormone-like substances, osteoclast activating factor, prostaglandins. Hypercalcemia is a feature in up to 8% of patients with bronchial carcinoma and the vast majority of these are found to have squamous cell tumours. This contrasts with other endocrine-related syndromes (e.g. ectopic Cushing's syndrome, syndrome of inappropriate antidiuretic hormone secretion) which are most commonly associated with small cell anaplastic lung cancer.

The clinical features of hypercalcaemia include anorexia, nausea, constipation, abdominal pain, polydipsia, polyuria, uraemia, hypokalaemia and mental changes ranging from confusion to coma. Neurological symptomatology often leads to a mistaken diagnosis of cerebral metastases, while the associated polydipsia and polyuria may also be confused with diabetes insipidus which occasionally complicates pituitary metastases. The syndrome remits following successful treatment of the primary tumour. Among inoperable patients medical management of hypercalcaemia often proves only partially successful, the serum calcium seldom falling into the normal range. Intravenous fluid replacement is the mainstay of treatment, specific hypocalcaemic therapy being necessary only if hypercalcaemia persists following rehydration. Such treatment may involve the use of high dose corticosteroids, phosphate, diphosphanates, mithramycin or calcitonin either singly or in combination.

Surgery remains the treatment of choice for squamous and other 'non-small cell' carcinomas of the bronchus, with a five year postoperative survival, in most series, of around 30% among patients with resectable disease. The outlook for patients with inoperable tumours is bleak with a median survival time after diagnosis of only five to six months. Performance status (an index of the patient's current physical status), weight loss and extent of disease are the main prognostic factors. A low performance status (immobility), weight loss greater than 10% of body weight in the previous six months and extrathoracic tumour spread all suggest a particularly poor prognosis.

Radical radiotherapy is capable of producing long term survival in a small proportion of cases, with a five year survival rate in highly selected patients of about 6%, but this approach is seldom possible owing to the severity of pre-existing lung disease (diminished pulmonary reserve greatly increases morbidity and mortality from radiation pneumonitis which invariably accompanies radical irradiation). Lower, palliative doses of radiotherapy are capable of producing worthwhile symptom control in a majority of patients but confer no survival advantage.

Certain chemotherapy combinations produce tumour responses in about 30-40% of patients with inoperable non-small cell lung cancer. These responses are usually only partial and relatively short-lived. Any survival advantage is likely to be small and there is continuing doubt surrounding the quality of life, as opposed to its quantity, in chemotherapy treated patients as compared to patients receiving supportive treatment only. Until more substantial evidence of therapeutic benefit is forthcoming existing drug combinations do not have a standard place in the management of inoperable non-small cell lung cancer.

Further reading

STEVENSON J. C. (1985) Malignant hypercalcaemia. *British Medical Journal*, **291**, 421.
GOLOMB H. M. (ed) (1983) Non-small cell carcinoma of the lung. *Seminars in Oncology*, **10**, 1.

Case 20

Answers

1. Bronchial asthma.
2. β-blockers increase airflow obstruction in asthmatic subjects and alternative anti-anginal therapy (calcium antagonist, nitrate) should be used.

Breathlessness is commonly the result of the combined influence of several individual causes, especially among elderly subjects. A positive outcome may not require that all factors are recognized and treated, but therapeutic success is unlikely unless the mechanism contributing most is correctly identified. In the case of Mrs Morson, there are obvious features of airflow obstruction but anaemia, obesity, cardiac failure and the space-occupying effect of a hiatus hernia are all potential contributory causes.

Impaired oxygen-carrying capacity in severe anaemic states places excessive demands on the circulation and the ventilatory apparatus. In general, however, chronic iron deficiency anaemia such as that due to severe oesophagitis, is not associated with impaired exercise performance unless the haemoglobin concentration is less than 8 g/dl. Gross obesity may produce a mild restrictive ventilatory defect with corresponding reductions in the compliance of the lungs and chest wall and some increase in the mechanical work of breathing. However, airflow obstruction is not a feature and while a moderate degree of obesity might contribute to impairment of effort tolerance it would not adequately explain nocturnal dyspnoea or wheeze. Furthermore, the absence of any recent increase in weight dictates against this being an important cause of Mrs Morson's new complaint. A diaphragmatic hernia is a rare cause of dyspnoea and is unlikely to be a major factor unless it is large and associated with an obvious abnormality on the chest X-ray.

Nocturnal attacks of dyspnoea suggest the possibilty of cardiac failure. Wheeze can also be a feature of left heart failure – so-called 'cardiac asthma' – and Mrs Morson's history of ischaemic heart disease, the ECG abnormality and the radiographic evidence of cardiomegaly are all in keeping with a possible cardiac cause for her symptoms. The failing heart may be dependent upon sympathetic drive and therapy with a β-blocker – in addition to its potential for increasing airflow obstruction in asthma and chronic bronchitis – can also precipitate cardiac decompensation in susceptible subjects. That this is not the correct explanation for Mrs Morson's symptoms is suggested by the absence of radiographic evidence of pulmonary oedema and the normal jugular venous pressure. It is the peak flow readings, however, which provide the most convincing evidence of an abnormality which primarily affects the intrapulmonary airways.

The hallmark of bronchial asthma is its variability with time and its reversibility in response to bronchodilator therapy. Most asthmatics show obvious diurnal variation with the lowest values for PEFR in the early morning (the 'morning dip'), an exaggeration of the normal circadian rhythm in airway calibre. In a proportion of asthmatics the nocturnal fall in PEFR is sufficient to cause the patient to wake, typically between 2.00 and 4.00 a.m. Such nocturnal attacks of asthma reflect poor overall control and severe bronchial lability, with amplitudes in peak flow rate of over 50% of the average daily value, are associated with an increased risk of ventilatory arrest and sudden death during recovery from acute attacks of asthma. The recognition of nocturnal symptoms is therefore very important and severely affected patients should be carefully monitored. Diurnal variation in airway calibre is also seen in chronic bronchitics but the amplitude of this variation is small compared to that in asthmatic subjects. The acute response to inhaled bronchodilator is also less marked (typically less than a 15% increase in PEFR or FEV_1). Although Mrs Morson had been a regular smoker, the degree of bronchial lability and reversibility following bronchodilator (31% increase in PEFR after salbutamol) clearly point to a diagnosis of bronchial asthma. It should be remembered, however, that asthma and chronic bronchitis are not mutually exclusive. As many as 30% of adult asthmatics will also satisfy the standard clinical criteria for chronic bronchitis.

The treatment of nocturnal asthma often proves difficult. Mild cases will frequently respond to improved overall control, e.g. from regular use of bronchodilator with or without additional anti-asthmatic medication through the day. More severe cases often respond only partially to combinations of sustained-release preparations of theopyllines and β-agonists which form the mainstay of treatment; inhaled anticholinergic therapy and topical corticosteroids are often disappointing. The use of a large dose of nebulized bronchodilator at bedtime or of a continuous subcutaneous infusion of a β-agonist offer alternative approaches, but nocturnal asthma may prove resistant to all of these measures and it continues to present an important therapeutic challenge.

A final point in Mrs Morson's case concerns the relation between gastro-oesophageal reflux and bronchial asthma. In some studies the frequency of hiatus hernia and radiological gastro-oesophageal reflux has been found to be significantly higher in asthmatic subjects compared to their frequency in age and sex matched controls. Other studies have suggested that asthmatic symptoms and PEFRs might be improved by medical anti-reflux treatments, cimetidine and surgical approaches aimed at restoring normal lower oesophageal function. The mechanism is poorly understood but is possibly mediated by a vagal reflex. Reflux oesophagitis might therefore represent a significant trigger for nocturnal symptoms ('gastric asthma'), especially among elderly subjects, and its successful treatment could make an important contribution to the control of the patient's asthma.

Further reading

COCHRANE, G. M. (1987) The difficult chronic asthmatic. *British Journal of Diseases of the Chest,* **81,** 313.
EDITORIAL. (1985) Gastric asthma? *Lancet,* **ii,** 1399.

Case 21

Answers

1. Desquamative interstitial pneumonitis – a variant of cryptogenic fibrosing alveolitis.
2. Initial therapy should consist of systemic corticosteroids (e.g. prednisolone 40-60 mg/day for 4–8 weeks).

Diffuse interstitial lung fibrosis is the common sequel to a wide variety of disease processes (e.g. pneumoconiosis, drug toxicity and hypersensitivity, extrinsic allergic alveolitis, radiation pneumonitis, sarcoidosis, uraemia, pulmonary venous hypertension, histiocytosis-X, tuberous sclerosis, lymphangioleiomyomatosis). In many cases, however, diffuse pulmonary fibrosis arises in the absence of any known cause. These cases of 'cryptogenic fibrosing alveolitis' are probably of varied aetiology but they tend to present a fairly uniform clinical and pathological picture. In about 35% of cases the same clinical picture occurs in association with a variety of 'connective tissue disorders'.

The onset of symptoms is usually insidious but it is common for patients to report that their illness developed in the aftermath of an influenza-like illness. Progressive exertional dyspnoea is commonly accompanied by an unproductive cough. Constitutional disturbances such as loss of appetite and weight loss occur frequently. Finger clubbing is a feature in about 60% of cases but the most consistent clinical finding is the presence of high-pitched, bilateral basal mid to late inspiratory lung crackles. In advanced cases crackles may be heard in early inspiration with tachypnoea, central cyanosis and signs of pulmonary hypertension and right heart failure. Radiologically the typical appearance consists of bilateral, predominantly basal, reticulo-nodular shadowing with middle and upper zone involvement as the disease progresses. In advanced disease, where there is considerable destruction of lung architecture, nodular shadows may be inconspicuous and widespread 'honeycomb' shadowing (due to groups of closely set ring shadows), most marked in the lung periphery, becomes the predominant feature. Fibrotic contraction of the lung parenchyma leads to progressive reduction in radiographic lung volume as a result of which the mediastinum may appear broadened.

The results of routine investigations are of little diagnostic value. A raised ESR and hyperglobulinaemia are common non-specific findings; circulating rheumatoid and antinuclear factors are often present even in the absence of associated autoimmune disorders. As with interstitial fibrosis due to other causes lung function tests characteristically reveal a restrictive defect with reduction of both total gas transfer and gas transfer coefficient. Lung volumes may be normal in the early stages of the disease when the most sensitive measure of impaired function is the demonstration of arterial oxygen desaturation following exercise.

Pathologically the early stages are characterized by an inflammatory exudate with mononuclear cell infiltration of the alveolar walls progressing to mural fibrosis (the term UIP – usual interstitial pneumonitis – is commonly applied in the North American literature). Progressive disease culminates in extensive fibrotic contraction of the lung and marked destruction and distortion of lung architecture, with widespread 'honeycombing' (due to bronchiolar dilatation and cyst formation) as the end-result. Desquamative interstitial pneumonitis (DIP) is recognized as a histological variant in which interstitial inflammation and fibrosis are less apparent and the dominant feature relates to the alveolar spaces which are uniformly crammed with mononuclear cells (alveolar macrophages). As a group, patients with DIP have a better prognosis than those with UIP. Patients with DIP generally show a favourable response to corticosteroids (overall, about 20% of patients with fibrosing alveolitis respond) and progression to end-stage lung disease is far less common than is the case with UIP. Other good prognostic features include a short duration of disease, younger age, presence of little established fibrosis in lung biopsies and rapid decline in lung function prior to treatment.

A therapeutic trial of treatment is indicated in all except elderly patients with stable disease. All clinical responses are evident within two months of starting treatment. The outlook is poor in non-responding patients but a trial of cyclophosphamide is probably worthwhile. About 50% of all patients are dead within 4–5 years. Death most commonly results from respiratory failure or cor pulmonale, often precipitated by respiratory infection. There is also a tenfold increase in deaths from lung cancer compared to a comparable control population (Turner-Warwick *et al.*, 1980).

Reference

TURNER-WARWICK, M., LEBOWITZ, M., BURROWS, B. and JOHNSON, A. (1980) Cryptogenic fibrosing alveoltis and lung cancer. *Thorax*, **35**, 496.

Case 22

Answers

1. There is an area of confluent consolidation in the left lower zone and a smaller, less well defined area of abnormal shadowing in the right upper zone.
2. Atypical pneumonia, probably caused by *Mycoplasma pneumoniae*.
3. Relevant investigations include:
   (a) Immunofluorescent antibody test for mycoplasma IgM antibody.

(b) Estimation of serum cold haemagglutinins.

(c) Complement fixation tests using paired sera collected about ten days apart. A single titre greater than 1:128 is highly suggestive of mycoplasma infection and a four-fold rise in titre between acute and convalescent sera is considered diagnostic.

(d) Culture of sputum and throat washings.

The vast majority of community–acquired pneumonias are caused by only a limited range of microbial agents. The spectrum of pathogens is far broader in nosocomial and opportunistic infections. In the community *Streptococcus pneumoniae* is by far the most common pathogen. By comparison, other bacterial causes are uncommon and gram-negative infections, in particular, are rare. *Staphylococcus aureus* plays an important role during influenza epidemics, while *Haemophilus influenzae* and *Branhamella catarrhalis* are important in patients with chronic bronchitis. Pneumonias due to *Legionella spp.* are well recognized but show marked geographic variation. Viral infection, most often *Influenza A*, is implicated in about 10–20% of cases and secondary bacterial infection commonly supervenes. About 15–20% of community–acquired pneumonias are the result of infection with *Mycoplasma pneumoniae, Coxiella burnetti* (causing Q fever) or *Chlamydia psittaci* (causing psittacosis), the latter two causes being much less common than mycoplasma infection. As a group these are often referred to as 'atypical' infections primarily in order to distinguish them from the more common bacterial pneumonias. In each case, however, the clinical illnesses bear a greater resemblance to viral infection although, in contrast to the latter, specific antimicrobial therapy is available.

Infections caused by *M. pneumoniae* appear to occur cyclically with the incidence peaking every three to five years. Clinical illness is most often apparent in children and young adults such that simultaneous cases occurring within a single household are not uncommon. Advancing age is not a barrier to infection, however, and the organism is often implicated in exacerbations of chronic bronchitis. An epidemic pattern is frequently recognized among closed populations, e.g. military recruits, schoolchildren, prisoners. The illness is generally benign and self-limiting but life-threatening pneumonic (lung abscesses, pneumatocoeles, adult respiratory distress syndrome) and extrapulmonary complications (see below) occur occasionally. Bronchiectasis, diffuse pulmonary fibrosis and Macleod's syndrome have all been described as late sequelae of mycoplasma infection.

The incubation period is about 14–21 days. Most infected individuals develop only mild upper or lower respiratory symptoms such as pharyngitis or bronchitis and only 3–10% of patients suffer clinically apparent pneumonia. The latter is frequently accompanied by symptoms of upper respiratory infection (25–50% of cases) as well as feverishness, malaise, and headaches. Cough is common and is usually unproductive. When sputum can be obtained – in about one third of cases – it is usually found to be mucoid, but mucopurulent and purulent sputum may also be produced. By contrast with pneumococcal pneumonia, haemoptysis and pleuritic chest pain are rare.

Typically, chest signs are relatively few – limited to localized wheezes and crackles without signs of consolidation – and radiographic changes disproportionately extensive. Bullous or haemorrhagic myringitis is infrequent in naturally occurring infection but, when present, should suggest the diagnosis. Other physical signs (cervical lymphadenopathy, tonsillar exudates, rashes, conjunctivitis and relative bradycardia) are encountered occasionally. Generalized lymphadenopathy and splenomegaly are unusual.

The chest X-ray typically shows patchy consolidation in one or other lower lobe, but bilateral abnormalities occur in 10–40% of cases. Lobar consolidation and pleural effusions are uncommon; hilar lymphadenopathy occurs occasionally and is commoner in children than in adults. X-ray changes, like clinical features, generally resolve within 10–21 days, but radiographic resolution sometimes takes several weeks.

Respiratory involvement is the primary feature of *M. pneumoniae* infection, psittacosis and Q-fever, but true systemic infection also occurs and each condition may be complicated by a wide range of extrapulmonary manifestations. Table A22.1 lists those that have been recognized in association with mycoplasma pneumonia. The range of possible clinical presentations is enormous and, as a result, mycoplasma infection will sometimes merit consideration in the differential diagnosis of multisystem disease.

Haemolytic anaemia is rare but is perhaps the best recognized of the extrapulmonary complications and, when present, characteristically occurs two to three weeks after the onset of the illness, coinciding with the peak cold agglutinin titre. Elevated cold haemagglutinins occur in about one half of all cases, but seldom result in more than subclinical haemolysis, producing a positive Coombs' test and a mild reticulocytosis. Only rarely is anaemia sufficient to warrant blood transfusion (warmed packed red cells) or treatment with systemic corticosteroids. In addition to Raynaud's phenomenon, one of the features shown by Mrs Robertson, the cold agglutinin response may also cause acrocyanosis, haemoglobinuria, renal failure, chronic cold haemagglutinin disease and even death from widespread thrombotic lesions.

Table A22.1 Extrapulmonary manifestations of *Mycoplasma pneumoniae* infections

Haematological: (see below)	Autoimmune haemolytic anaemia, thrombocytopenia (see below) disseminated intravascular coagulation.
Musculoskeletal: ($\sim$ 40%)	Myalgia, arthralgia, polyarthritis.
Neurological: ($\sim$ 5%)	Aseptic meningitis, meningoencephalitis, cranial and peripheral neuropathy, cerebellar ataxia, transverse myelitis.
Dermatological: ($\sim$ 25%)	Macular rash, erythema nodosum, erythema multiforme, Stevens-Johnson syndrome.
Gastrointestinal: ($\sim$ 10–45%)	Gastroenteritis, hepatitis, pancreatitis.
Cardiac: ($\sim$ 5%)	Pericarditis, myocarditis, conduction defects.
Miscellaneous:	Glomerulonephritis, interstitial nephritis, generalized lymphadenopathy, splenomegaly.

It is important to remember that elevated cold agglutinin titres are not diagnostic of mycoplasma infection. They may be seen in association with lymphoproliferative disorders, *idiopathic* chronic cold haemagglutinin disease, connective tissue disorders and a variety of other infections (e.g. adenovirus, influenza, CMV, mumps, syphilis, malaria, Legionnaires' disease), but especially infectious mononucleosis (also a rare cause of pneumonia) which would have entered the clinical differential diagnosis in the present case.

While the diagnosis of mycoplasma pneumonia may be suspected on clinical grounds, confirmation is usually retrospective and reliant upon serological results. Isolation of the organism is difficult and may take one or more weeks. The most useful diagnostic test is the immunofluorescent test for mycoplasma IgM antibody. This is both sensitive ($\sim$ 75%) and highly specific and is positive early enough – within a few days of the onset of illness – to be useful clinically and to influence choice of treatment.

Therapy with erythromycin or tetracycline (contraindicated in children under eight years) for 10–14 days hastens resolution of the clinical features and radiographic abnormalities. During epidemic years the frequency of mycoplasma infection is such as to warrant routine use of erythromycin along with a semi-synthetic penicillin (usually amoxycillin or ampicillin) as first-line treatment of community-acquired pneumonias. During influenza epidemics, or when pneumonia due to *Staphylococcus aureus* is suspected clinically, flucloxacillin should be included in the initial choice of antibiotic therapy.

Further reading

RESEARCH COMMITTEE OF THE BRITISH THORACIC SOCIETY AND THE PUBLIC HEALTH LABORATORY SERVICE (1987) Community-acquired pneumonia in adults in British hospitals in 1982–1983: a survey of aetiology, mortality, prognostic factors and outcome. *Quarterly Journal of Medicine*, **62**, 195.

ALI, N. J., SILLIS, M., ANDREWS, B. E. *et al.* (1986) The clinical spectrum and diagnosis of *Mycoplasma pneumoniae* infection. *Quarterly Journal of Medicine*, **58**, 241.

Case 23

Answers

1. There has been a major dehiscence of the pneumonectomy stump resulting in a bronchopleural fistula.
2. The patient should be nursed on his left side in order to minimize further entry of fluid from the left hemithorax into the bronchial tree. Closed intercostal drainage of the pneumonectomy space and broad spectrum antibiotic therapy should be instituted and the patient referred back to the thoracic surgeons for further management of the bronchopleural fistula.

Surgery remains the treatment of choice for early, localized carcinoma of the bronchus and, having established the diagnosis, clinical evaluation of the patient serves two purposes:

1. To establish the extent of spread of disease,
2. To determine the patient's physiological fitness for pulmonary resection.

Ultimately, early postoperative morbidity and mortality as well as long term survival are dependent upon the care used in the selection of patients for surgical treatment. The operative mortality rate will vary between about 4% and 10% whilst 5–15% of patients will experience major complications. Increasing age, restricted pulmonary reserve and pneumonectomy (as opposed to less extensive resection) are recognized as high-risk factors.

The most common postoperative complications are either cardiac (arrythmias, myocardial infarction, cardiac failure) or respiratory in origin. With improvements in preoperative assessment respiratory failure due to loss of functioning lung tissue – at one time the cause of about 40% of operative deaths – is no longer a common problem. Bronchopulmonary infection, pulmonary embolism and pleural empyema all occur more frequently. The development of a bronchopleural fistula is an infrequent but serious complication of pneumonectomy and because it may occur 'late' and present as a medical emergency physicians should be familiar with its clinical manifestations.

Following pneumonectomy the pleural cavity initially contains air but subsequently begins to fill with serosanguinous fluid. The pneumonectomy space is generally completely filled, and uniformly radio-opaque within 2–4 months of surgery. In the early postoperative period therefore an air-fluid level is to be expected in the ipsilateral hemithorax. Disruption of the pneumonectomy stump results in a direct communication between the pleural cavity and the bronchial tree when fluid from the pneumonectomy space is allowed to enter the airway and soil the contralateral lung. A major dehiscence such as that seen in Mr McLeod produces sudden onset of dyspnoea with expectoration of large amounts of pleural fluid and a fall in the level of fluid on the plain chest X-ray. Flooding of the airway causes marked hypoxia and circulatory collapse soon follows. Confusion with other respiratory emergencies is unlikely provided that the condition is borne in mind.

A post-pneumonectomy bronchopleural fistula represents a unique situation where the pleural cavity is filled with fluid. In the absence of surgical interference the clinical picture is quite different and depends primarily upon the magnitude of the air leak. Used strictly the term bronchopleural fistula applies to a communication between the pleural cavity and the bronchial tree but it is sometimes applied to any communication between the pleural cavity and the lung, including an alveolar leak. A leak at alveolar level results in a pneumothorax with pulmonary collapse and displacement of the mediastinum to the affected side. The amount of air escaping from the lung periphery is generally small such that, when pleural drainage is established, alveolar ventilation is not compromised to any significant extent. Even if mechanical ventilation is undertaken the leak is seldom increased sufficiently to prevent adequate alveolar ventilation. By contrast a communication between a major bronchus and the pleural space (e.g. following traumatic bronchial rupture) will result in severe respiratory insufficiency because the air leak is large relative to the tidal volume and tension builds up rapidly within the pleural cavity. Alveolar ventilation in this setting is inadequate and is not improved by positive pressure ventilation which only serves to increase the air leak. Urgent management requires endotracheal intubation in order to isolate the fistula and intercostal tube drainage followed by thoracotomy and primary repair of the bronchopleural fistula.

Further reading

EDITORIAL (1984) The staging of lung cancer. *Thorax*, **39**, 401.

Case 24

Answers

1. Cryptogenic pulmonary eosinophilia.
2. Treatment is with systemic steroids which typically results in rapid resolution of clinical and radiographic abnormalities.

The term pulmonary eosinophilia is applied to a group of diverse conditions that are characterized by abnormal radiographic lung shadows and accompanying peripheral blood eosinophilia (eosinophils $> 0.5 \times 10^9$/l). A simple descriptive classification was proposed by Crofton *et al.* (1952), but our understanding of pulmonary eosinophilia has progressed to the point where a more useful classification can be based upon aetiology (Table A24.1).

Table A24.1 Causes of pulmonary eosinophilia (PE)

Fungal hypersensitivity
Especially due to *Aspergillus fumigatus* (80% of all cases of PE in the UK), *Candida albicans*

Heminthic infestation
e.g. Ascariasis, filariasis, schistosomiasis, toxocariasis

Drug hypersensitivity
Especially nitrofurantoin, PAS, sulphonamides

Idiopathic
Associated with pulmonary vasculitis (Wegener's granulomatosis, Churg–Strauss syndrome
Associated with systemic vasculitis (polyarteritis nodosa)
No associated vasculitis: cryptogenic PE or chronic eosinophilic pneumonia (see text)

Miscellaneous
e.g. Hypereosinophilic syndrome, PE associated with Hodgkin's disease, carcinoma

---

On a worldwide basis the most common cause of pulmonary eosinophilia is parasitic infestation, most often with microfilaria when the term tropical eosinophilia is often applied. Endemic areas include India, Pakistan and Southeast Asia where the typical patient is a young adult with insidious onset of cough, wheeze and dyspnoea associated with febrile symptoms and weight loss. The chest X-ray usually shows diffuse mottling or miliary opacities. The diagnosis rests upon the demonstration of elevated antifilarial antibody titres. Other infestations produce a similar clinical picture, but patients are more often asymptomatic. Diagnosis requires the demonstration of ova, larvae or adult worms in the patient's stool or, in the case of Toxocara ('visceral larva migrans'), where organisms are not demonstrable, the detection of serum antibodies.

In the UK pulmonary eosinophilia is most commonly encountered as a manifestation of drug hypersensitivity, as a complication of bronchial asthma due to fungal hypersensitivity or, more rarely, in association with vasculitis or neoplasia. However, none of these explanations apply here. The history fails to suggest an obvious candidate for drug hypersensitivity and there are no clear clinical pointers toward a diagnosis of underlying malignancy. Nor are there any features of a systemic vasculitis and certainly none of the usual clinical accompaniments of either Churg–Strauss syndrome (history of atopic diseases, especially allegic rhinitis, extrathoracic involvement) or Wegener's granulomatosis (nasal discharge, sinusitis, glomerulonephritis).

Whilst asthmatic symptoms are present there are no features of fungal hypersensitivity and specifically no evidence of allergic bronchopulmonary aspergillosis (ABPA) – the cause of about 80% of all cases of asthmatic pulmonary eosinophilia in the UK. ABPA is most often encountered in atopic (skin test positive, 'extrinsic') asthmatics. Less commonly it may also complicate late onset (skin test negative, 'intrinsic') asthma, but the negative skin prick test to *Aspergillus fumigatus* and the normal serum total IgE level, characteristically markedly raised in ABPA, serve to exclude this diagnosis. Nasal polyposis and peripheral blood eosinophilia are both common features of skin test negative, late onset asthma, but other findings in this case – markedly raised ESR, weight loss, distinctive radiographic appearances – point to more than a simple, uncomplicated case of bronchial asthma.

Within the idiopathic group of pulmonary eosinophilias, those cases showing no evidence of vasculitis tend to form a well defined population with distinct clinical, radiological and immunological features. These cases of cryptogenic pulmonary eosinophilia (CPE) are characterized pathologically by an interstitial and intra-alveolar infiltrate consisting primarily of eosinophils but also including some chronic inflammatory cells. The term 'chronic eosinophilic pneumonia' has been applied (Carrington *et al.*, 1969). Immunologically, the most notable feature is a normal or only slightly raised serum total IgE level with a disproportionately marked eosinophilia. The contrasting immunological findings in parasitic infestation (marked increases in both eosinophils and total IgE) and fungal hypersensitivity, e.g. ABPA (relatively mild eosinophilia in relation to markedly elevated total IgE) suggest the operation of different aetiological agents and the existence of CPE as a distinct entity.

Most patients with CPE are non-atopic. The clinical presentation is usually with cough, dyspnoea and prominent systemic manifestations (malaise, weight loss, fever, night sweats, grossly raised ESR, anaemia). Asthmatic features are present in about half of the cases. The radiographic changes are virtually pathognomonic (Figure 24.1) – dense areas of peripheral, non-segmental,

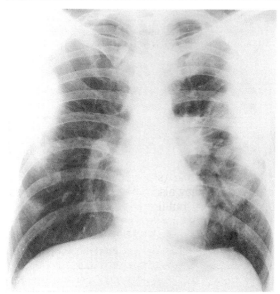

Figure A24.1 Cryptogenic pulmonary eosinophilia: bilateral, symmetrical peripheral homogeneous consolidation–'photographic negative' of pulmonary oedema

homogeneous consolidation with ill-defined margins. The appearances have been likened to a 'photographic negative' (or reverse appearance) of the 'bat's wing' shadows of pulmonary oedema (Gaensler and Carrington, 1977).

Rapid clinical and radiographic resolution follows treatment with modest doses of systemic corticosteroids (e.g. prednisolone, 20 mg daily). Unlike ABPA which gives rise to a characteristic form of bronchiectasis involving the central airways, pulmonary infiltrates in CPE resolve without evidence of bronchial damage. Recurrent pulmonary infiltration may arise several years after discontinuation of therapy. Responsiveness to steroids is retained, however, and the long term outlook for affected patients is good.

References and further reading

CARRINGTON, C. B., ADDINGTON, W. W., GOFF, A. M. *et al.*, (1969) Chronic eosinophilic pneumonia. *The New England Journal of Medicine*, **280**, 787.

GAENSLER, E. A. and CARRINGTON, C. B. (1977) Peripheral opacities in chronic eosinophilic pneumonia: the photographic negative of pulmonary oedema. *American Journal of Roentgenology*, **128**, 1.

TURNER-WARWICK, M., ASSEM, E. S. K. and LOCKWOOD, M. (1976) Cryptogenic pulmonary eosinophilia. *Clinical Allergy*, **6** 135.

Case 25

Answers

1. It is most likely that Mrs Sales' 'laryngeal wheeze' is the result of a functional disorder of the larynx associated with underlying psychiatric abnormality.
2. Bronchoscopy or laryngoscopy during an attack of wheeze will suggest the diagnosis if the vocal cords are seen to be adducted throughout the respiratory cycle.

'Not all that wheezes is bronchial asthma', (Proctor, 1983). Wheeze is also a feature of other disorders associated with diffuse narrowing of intrapulmonary airways (chronic obstructive bronchitis, emphysema and bronchiectasis). Localized bronchial obstruction due to a bronchial adenoma (see Answer 5) or bronchial carcinoma may also generate wheeze, usually monophonic and localized and therefore clinically distinguishable from the multiple and diffusely distributed wheezes of bronchial asthma. A similar situation can arise following foreign body inhalation which, more commonly in children than in adults, may occur in the absence of any clear history of aspiration. A chest radiograph in full expiration will usually help to confirm the diagnosis when it shows localized air trapping ('obstructive' emphysema) due to a ball-valve effect of the foreign body. Bronchoscopy is essential when any diagnostic doubt remains. In children cystic fibrosis may present with wheeze in association with recurrent lower respiratory infection. The presence of radiographic changes (upper lobe fibrosis, bronchiectasis) and the absence of, or only minor changes in, the diurnal variation in peak expiratory flow rate (marked diurnal variation is characteristic of asthma) will help to identify these children.

Upper airway obstruction due to laryngeal or tracheal lesions typically causes a loud wheeze of single pitch, clinically recognizable as stridor, but in practice the sound that is produced may closely resemble that seen in asthma (see Answer 18). Diagnostic difficulty may also arise, especially among elderly patients, when wheezing is a prominent presenting feature of left heart failure – so-called 'cardiac asthma' – when airways obstruction is secondary to bronchial mucosal oedema. Associated clinical signs of low cardiac output, pulsus alternans, a third heart sound, raised jugular venous pressure, ECG abnormalties and radiological signs of pulmonary venous congestion or pulmonary oedema will generally serve to differentiate from asthma of bronchial origin.

Mrs Sales' case demonstrates yet another potential source of diagnostic confusion. Here a functional laryngeal disorder was initially misdiagnosed as bronchial asthma. The literature contains many similar reports of patients who have been variously diagnosed as having 'paradoxical vocal cord movement', 'factitious asthma', 'emotional laryngeal wheezing', 'vocal cord dysfunction', 'Munchausen's stridor' or 'adult spasmodic croup'. In all of these cases vocal cord malfunction has been either suspected or confirmed (by laryngoscopy) as the cause of respiratory symptoms. During attacks the vocal cords are seen to be closely adducted. Different clinical features and hence different diagnoses and terminologies have been applied depending upon which phase of the respiratory cycle has been most affected. Bronchial asthma is most closely simulated when the cords are adducted during both inspiration and expiration. The majority of cases have been described in young adult females in whom there is a strong association with underlying emotional problems. It has been suggested that the syndrome represents a form of hysterical conversion disorder. Incorrect diagnosis, usually bronchial asthma, has often led to inappropriate treatment applied over prolonged periods without therapeutic benefit.

Often the clinical history will yield useful clues to the presence of psychological problems. Mrs Sales' tragic medical history with enforced retirement on health grounds and her earlier depressive illness all suggest the possibility of emotional conflict. Clinically, the finding of inspiratory and/or expiratory noises with maximum intensity over the larynx – and transmission to the chest with diminishing intensity over the peripheral lung fields – points to a laryngeal source of wheeze rather than the intrapulmonary airways. Furthermore, the presence of a normal arterial $P\text{co}_2$ would not be expected during an acute attack of asthma when one would also expect to see radiographic evidence of hyperinflation. Mrs Sales had a normal chest X-ray.

During asymptomatic periods pulmonary function tests and endoscopic examination of the upper airway show no abnormality, clearly pointing to a functional rather than an organic cause for the disorder. The diagnosis is confirmed, however, when the typical glottic abnormality is observed during a symptomatic episode. In common with organic causes of upper airway obstruction symptoms are relieved by the inhalation of a mixture of helium and

138

oxygen. Definitive treatment centres around the use of speech therapy and psychiatric counselling which are often associated with dramatic clinical responses. The outlook for most patients is favourable, the majority being rendered asymptomatic within 12 months.

References and further reading

PROCTOR, D. F. (1983) All that wheezes . . . . *American Review of Respiratory Disease*, **127**, 261.
CHRISTOPHER, K. L., WOOD, R. P., ECKERT, R. C. *et al.* (1983) Vocal-cord dysfunction presenting as asthma. *The New England Journal of Medicine*, **308**, 1566.

Case 26

Answers

1. Motor neurone disease.
2. Severe bilateral diaphragmatic weakness.
3. Fluoroscopic screening will usually show reduced diaphragmatic movement but can be unreliable. Measurement of transdiaphragmatic pressure using gastric and oesophageal balloons will provide more direct confirmation of the diagnosis. This is unnecessary when the clinical features and results of simple tests of lung function point unequivocally to diaphragmatic weakness.

Orthopnoea is a symptom classically associated with cardiac failure. It is less well recognized that severe orthopnoea can also be the result of diaphragmatic weakness or paralysis. Clinically, this possibility is easily overlooked. In the recumbent position the weight of the abdominal viscera pushes the weak or paralysed diaphragm high into the thorax, compressing the lower lobes with the resulting posture related symptoms of dyspnoea and tachypnoea and radiographic evidence of basal atelectasis. Respiratory muscle weakness also produces a change in the pattern of breathing with jerkiness of respiratory movements and asynchrony between the chest and abdomen (normally movements are smooth and synchronous, e.g. the chest and abdomen moving outward together during inspiration). With severe diaphragmatic weakness there is often marked abdominal paradox, when the abdomen appears to be sucked inward during inspiration.

Respiratory muscle weakness is a feature of a wide variety of neuromuscular disorders (Table A26.1). In motor neurone disease, respiratory infection and failure are common terminal events and respiratory muscle weakness is the rule in symptomatic patients. Severe diaphragmatic weakness usually parallels severe weakness in other muscle groups. In some cases early and preferential involvement of the anterior horn cells of the phrenic nerve nucleus results in an early onset of respiratory muscle weakness and this subsequently dominates the clinical picture. In about 1–5% of patients the initial presentation is with respiratory symptoms, the more typical features of amyotrophic lateral sclerosis and bulbar involvement usually appearing soon afterwards. In Mr MacCutcheon's case, the presence of hoarseness due to weakness affecting the extrinsic muscles of the larynx, muscle fasiculation and the distribution of weakness and wasting in the absence of abnormal sensory signs all served to suggest motor neurone disease. This diagnosis was subsequently confirmed by electromyography.

Table A26.1   Neuromuscular syndromes producing respiratory muscle weakness

Cervical spinal cord injuries: high (C1,C2) and mid cord (C3-C5) injuries produce diaphragmatic paresis; lower cervical (C7,C8) and upper thoracic (T1–T6) cord injuries affect intercostal and abdominal muscles, impairing cough but not ventilation

Anterior horn cell injury e.g. poliomyelitis, motor neurone disease (amyotrophic lateral sclerosis, Kugelberg–Welander syndrome, Werdnig–Hoffman syndrome)

Peripheral neuropathy, e.g. Guillain-Barré syndrome

Disorders of the neuro-muscular junction, e.g. myasthenia gravis

Muscular dystrophies

Myotonic dystrophy (dystrophia myotonica)

Myopathic disorders e.g. polymyositis, myopathies secondary to undernutrition, alcohol, steroids, specific enzyme deficiencies – acid maltase deficiency

Idiopathic diaphragmatic paralysis

As with poliomyelitis both the spinal and medullary motor neurones are affected in amyotrophic lateral sclerosis. Because the clinical picture is dominated by the effects of muscle weakness the effect of medullary involvement on respiratory function is uncertain. In the absence of significant diaphragmatic weakness, reduction in vital capacity (VC) is often associated with a considerable increase in residual volume. The total lung capacity is often relatively normal even when there is quite severe generalized muscle weakness.

When there is severe diaphragmatic weakness in the absence of major weakness affecting other muscle groups, as with Mr MacCutcheon, lung volumes may be near normal in the upright position but a marked fall in VC is seen in the supine posture. In normal subjects the fall should be less than 25%; in patients with diaphragmatic paralysis the fall in VC has been reported to be in the range, 35–97%. Carbon dioxide retention is common but is often unsuspected when the VC in the upright position is relatively well preserved. In the early stages patients develop respiratory failure only during sleep when hypoventilation is most marked. The flow volume loop shows characteristic flattening of the inspiratory limb – a pattern also seen in pulmonary restriction and upper airway obstruction. Whereas the K_{co} is low in patients with pulmonary restriction, it is often raised in extrapulmonary restriction and this combination of abnormalities is sufficient to suggest that the diaphragm should be screened under load.

Amyotrophic lateral sclerosis (ALS) carries a poor prognosis, death resulting from bulbar failure. Chronic spinal muscular atrophy of adults (Kugelberg–Welander syndrome) affects only lower motor neurones and carries a better prognosis than ALS but diaphragmatic involvement and ventilatory failure may occur. There are no known treatments that will alter the natural history of motor neurone disease. However, various forms of breathing aid may be appropriate for symptomatic relief in selected patients, e.g. in the treatment of distressing orthopnoea. When the VC is moderately impaired this might be achieved by nocturnal support using a Rocking Bed. With more severe impairment more effective support is derived from negative pressure ventilation using a Cuirass Shell. When diaphragmatic paralysis occurs in the absence of generalized neuromuscular disease (idiopathic diaphragmatic paralysis), diaphragmatic pacing offers an effective method of treatment.

Further reading

NEWSOM-DAVIS, J., GOLDMAN, M., LOH, L. and CASSON, M. (1976) Diaphragm function and alveolar hypoventilation. *Quarterly Journal of Medicine*, **45**, 87.

NIGHTINGALE, S., BATEMAN, D., BATES, D. *et al.* (1982) Enigmatic dyspnoea. *Lancet*, **1**, 933.

Case 27

Answers

1. Adult respiratory distress syndrome.
2. The prognosis is poor with a mortality rate of about 60%.
3. Treatment includes intermittent positive pressure ventilation using a positive end-expiratory pressure, with the aim of keeping the $Pa_{O_2} > 7.99\,kPa$.

The clinical syndrome of adult respiratory distress syndrome (ARDS, 'shock lung') is readily recognizable when a patient with previously normal lungs develops pulmonary oedema and refractory hypoxaemia against a background of some predisposing insult (Table A27.1). It is characteristic of ARDS that a latent period of between 4 and 24 hours follows the underlying trigger before respiratory symptoms and hypoxaemia become apparent. Dyspnoea and tachycardia are the main clinical findings. Sputum and signs of respiratory infection are common late complications and, in the early stages, cough is usually unproductive. Central cyanosis may be apparent despite a high inspired oxygen concentration. Abnormal chest signs are absent at the outset; widespread crackles and wheezes appear over the course of 24–48 hours. A wide variety of additional extra-pulmonary features (renal failure, liver failure, CNS depression, hypotension, metabolic abmormalities such as hypoalbuminaemia and metabolic acidosis) are often associated with ARDS, reflecting the systemic nature of the initial insult. Respiratory infection and tension pneumothorax (a manifestation of barotrauma in ventilated patients) are important complications.

Initially the chest radiograph is normal. The earliest changes of interstitial oedema progress over 24–48 hours to diffuse, bilateral

Table A27.1 Clinical criteria for diagnosis of adult respiratory distress syndrome

Presence of appropriate risk factor, e.g. trauma, sepsis, pancreatitis, haemorrhagic shock
Progressive respiratory failure with severe hypoxaemia
Radiographic evidence of pulmonary oedema
Previously normal lungs
Absence of cardiac failure

confluent areas of consolidation showing an alveolar filling pattern. Such pulmonary oedema – the result of increased pulmonary microvascular permeability – constitutes the hallmark of ARDS and is the cause of the reduced lung compliance that characterizes the condition. The radiographic changes, like the clinical features, are entirely non-specific and essentially the same as those due to pulmonary oedema secondary to increased intravascular hydrostatic pressure. In an elderly patient with a previous history of ischaemic heart disease left heart failure must obviously be considered in the differential diagnosis. Differentiation may prove difficult on clinical grounds alone but pulsus alternans, third or fourth heart sounds and raised central venous pressure will point to a cardiac cause. The radiographic features may also help. Raised pulmonary venous pressure results in upper lobe vein diversion of blood and radiographically visible dilatation of upper lobe veins. Pleural effusions are also a common accompaniment of pulmonary venous hypertension, but are rarely the result of increased vascular permeability other than in the presence of pneumonia, chest trauma or pericarditis. Cardiomegaly is not a feature of ARDS, but Mrs Hammond was known to have a degree of cardiac enlargement prior to the onset of respiratory symptoms. In these circumstances, Swan–Ganz catheterization with measurement of indirect left atrial pressure will remove any doubt about the aetiology of pulmonary oedema. Hydrostatic pulmonary oedema is generally associated with a pulmonary capillary wedge pressure greater than 2.66 kPa. Normal values (0.66–1.60 kPa) would be expected in ARDS.

After vigorous treatment directed towards the underlying cause the management of ARDS is essentially supportive. Adequate arterial oxygenation requires mechanical ventilation with the use of a positive end-expiratory pressure (5–10 cm H_2O) and high inspired oxygen concentrations. Other methods of ventilation (e.g. high frequency jet ventilation, high frequency positive pressure ventilation) have been suggested as a means of reducing pulmonary barotrauma, but none has been shown to have any clear advantage over conventional techniques. More specific therapy aimed at reducing pulmonary microvascular permeability has been attempted with corticosteroids, β_2 agonists and prostaglandins, but none of these approaches is of conclusive benefit. The use of steroids, in particular, has been called into question following a recent study in which their prophylactic use in a group of patients at high risk of ARDS was associated with increased mortality due to infection. Despite earlier recognition of the problem and improvements in intensive care the mortality remains very high, averaging 60%. Severe and persistent respiratory dysfunction, sepsis and multiple organ failure portend a particularly poor outlook.

Further reading

EDITORIAL (1987) The adult respiratory distress syndrome – 20 years on. *Thorax*, **42**, 641.

Case 28

Answers

1. Tuberculosis.
2. A positive *tuberculin test* supports the diagnosis but definitive confirmation rests upon positive bacteriological findings. *Pleural biopsy* should be carried out in conjunction with diagnostic pleural aspiration as a part of the investigation of any pleural effusion unless there is a bleeding tendency or an empyema is present. If tuberculosis is suspected both tissue and fluid should be submitted for culture; needle biopsies of the pleura yield histological evidence of tuberculous granulation tissue in about 70–80% of cases. When sputum is unobtainable, *bronchoscopy* with microscopy and culture of bronchial aspirate may be diagnostic. Occasionally, confirmation may be obtained from characteristic histological changes in *transbronchial lung biopsies*. In bacteriologically negative cases a clear response to a *therapeutic trial of antituberculous chemotherapy* offers reliable clinical confirmation of the diagnosis.

The diagnosis of a rheumatoid pleural effusion is primarily one of exclusion. There are no pathognomonic features and other conditions, tuberculosis in particular, may be closely mimicked. In Mr Provan's case the diagnosis of tuberculosis was established from pleural biopsies, histological sections of which showed scanty acid-alcohol fast bacilli; bronchial aspirate was also positive on direct smear. However, on clinical grounds alone – Mr Provan's relative youth (see below), his history of malaise and fever and the apical radiographic changes with cavitation – tuberculosis would appear the most likely explanation.

As with most of the pleuropulmonary complications of rheumatoid disease, pleural effusions occur more commonly in men than in women (M:F ratio about 4:1) and usually in association with seropositive disease. Mr Provan certainly satisfies these criteria but, in general, rheumatoid pleurisy is very uncommon under the age of 45. Although moderate or large effusions are seen occasionally in association with rheumatoid disease, they are typically small and asymptomatic. Systemic upset, in particular, is unusual unless secondary infection is present.

The pleural fluid is usually pale or dark yellow and may appear opalescent. Occasionally a high fat content produces a pseudochylous effusion and, rarely, the effusion appears purulent (empyema) but is sterile on culture. The fluid is an exudate (protein content > 30 g/l) often with an elevated level of lactic acid dehydrogenase (LDH) and a low sugar content (< 1.65 mmol/l). The latter is also a feature of infection, however, and raised LDH levels may be a feature of any chronic effusion. The presence of rheumatoid factor in the pleural fluid is similarly unhelpful as it may also appear in effusions without a rheumatoid aetiology. The cellular content is variable, some effusions showing a predominance of lymphocytes, others a predominance of neutrophils. There are therefore no diagnostic features. Pleural biopsies too generally yield non-specific histological changes and only rarely will they show any diagnostic features (rheumatoid necrobiosis).

Intrapulmonary rheumatoid nodules generally present as rounded, well defined homogeneous opacities. They are usually about 1–2 cm in diameter and may be either single or multiple. A number of closely grouped rheumatoid nodules might produce an area of 'patchy' radiographic shadowing, but this would be an unlikely explanation for the X-ray abnormality in this case. Lung nodules are usually symptomless but may cavitate and rupture into a bronchus producing a small haemoptysis or they may become secondarily infected. Rarely, a subpleural nodule will rupture into the pleural cavity producing a bronchopleural fistula and a resulting hydropneumothorax.

Table A28.1 lists the other recognized pleuropulmonary manifestations of rheumatoid disease. Rheumatoid fibrosing alveolitis usually arises in patients with established arthritis but, in a small proportion of patients, clinical and/or radiographic features of pulmonary fibrosis precede joint changes. Clinically significant lung involvement is uncommon (about 1% of patients), males exceeeding females in a ratio of 2:1. A much higher proportion of patients, especially those with severe arthritis, will show restrictive abnormalities of lung function or autopsy evidence of pulmonary fibrosis. The natural history of the condition and its response to treatment are similar to 'cryptogenic' fibrosing alveolitis (see Answer 21).

Table A28.1 Pleuropulmonary complications of rheumatoid disease

Pleural effusion
Pleural adhesions; thickened pleura
Hydropneumothorax (secondary to ruptured subpleural nodule)
Fibrosing alveolitis
Caplan's syndrome (rheumatoid pneumoconiosis)
Obliterative bronchiolitis
Intrapulmonary nodules
Pulmonary hypertension (rare, secondary to pulmonary vascular involvement)
Increased incidence of respiratory infections

Caplan's syndrome refers to the development of fibrotic lung nodules in patients with rheumatoid arthritis and coalworker's pneumoconiosis. The condition is not confined to coalworkers, however, and may occur in association with other pneumoconioses including asbestosis. The nodules usually arise in crops and show histological features of both necrobiotic nodules and the lesions of progressive massive fibrosis. Its pathogenesis is poorly understood but it would appear that the presence of mineral dust in the lung modifies the immunopathological response to rheumatoid factor.

Although it is not recognized as a characteristic feature of rheumatoid disease as many as 30% of patients will show physiological evidence of small airways obstruction. That this is not simply smoking-related is suggested by the rare development in some rheumatoid patients of rapidly progressive air flow obstruction due to an obliterative bronchiolitis. In one series this complication proved rapidly fatal, despite treatment, in five out of six affected patients (Geddes *et al.* 1977). Rarely, pulmonary hypertension develops in the absence of gross pulmonary fibrosis or airways disease when it is secondary to pulmonary vascular involvement by the rheumatoid process.

Further reading

GEDDES, D. M., CORRIN, B., BREWERTON, D. A. *et al.* (1977) Progressive airways obliteration in adults and its association with rheumatoid disease. *Quarterly Journal of Medicine*, **184**, 427.

TURTON, C. W. G. (1987) Troublesome pleural fluid. *British Journal of Diseases of the Chest*, **81**, 217.

146

Case 29

Answers

1. The main differential diagnosis lies between opportunistic infection and drug-induced pulmonary toxicity. Other less likely possibilities also needing to be considered are lymphomatous infiltration, pulmonary oedema and pulmonary haemorrhage.
2. Bleomycin is a well recognized cause of pulmonary toxicity. Among the other agents given to Mr Pottinger, both procarbazine and vincristine have also been implicated, albeit only rarely.

Radiographic pulmonary infiltration arising during the course of treatment for malignant disease presents a not uncommon clinical diagnostic problem. The radiographic appearances are often relatively non-specific and the usual clinical findings and functional abnormalities – cough, dyspnoea, hypoxaemia, restrictive ventilatory defect, impaired gas transfer – are similar for the various possible causes.

Pulmonary haemorrhage is an unlikely explanation in the absence of severe thrombocytopenia (platelet count $< 10 \times 10^9/l$) and this typically produces an increased gas transfer coefficient (K_{co}) rather than the reverse as in this case. Lung involvement has been reported in as many as 43% of patients with Hodgkin's disease, but there was no evidence of this when Mr Pottinger first presented and pulmonary disease progression would be most improbable when there is evidence of a good therapeutic response at other sites. Furthermore, the radiographic pattern (diffuse 'alveolar' shadowing) is not one that is associated with malignant infiltration: lung involvement in Hodgkin's disease is usually the result of direct spread along perivascular and peribronchial lymphatics from enlarged hilar and mediastinal lymph nodes; less often haematogenous dissemination produces discrete peripheral opacities or, rarely, 'miliary' mottling. Although the reported X-ray abnormality is consistent with pulmonary oedema the absence of other features of cardiac failure and its subacute onset are against this diagnosis. It is worthy of note, however, that non-cardiogenic pulmonary oedema has been described as a rare acute complication of therapy with a number of cytotoxic drugs (cyclophosphamide, methotrexate, VM-26, cytosine arabinoside).

In addition to the neutropenic and lymphopenic effects of cytotoxic therapy Hodgkin's patients also suffer impaired cellular immune responses and are particularly susceptible to infections caused by facultative intracellular parasites such as *Mycobacterium tuberculosis* and *Cryptococcus neoformans.* However, the risk of infection in patients with malignant lymphomas, as with leukaemias and solid tumours, is most closely related to neutropenia. A close inverse correlation is seen between the the severity of neutropenia and the risk of infection: nadir neutrophil counts less than $0.1 \times 10^9/l$ have been associated with an infective risk of about 30%, compared with a 2% risk if the neutrophil count remains above $2 \times 10^9/l$. Among fatal infections in patients treated for malignant lymphoma by far the highest proportion are due to bacteria (86%), with fungi (13%), protozoa (0.6%) and viruses (0.3%) accounting for progressively fewer infective deaths. Pneumonia and septicaemia are the most common types of infection and for pneumonic infections gram-negative bacilli and fungi are the usual pathogens. These patients are generally acutely and severely ill and yet they often fail to show the typical features of pneumonia: cough and sputum are commonly absent and radiographic consolidation may be inconspicuous or absent in the early stages of the illness. Infection with the protozoan parasite, *Pneumocystis carinii,* often has a more insidious onset and may be suspected on clinical grounds when extensive, bilateral 'alveolar' consolidation is associated with tachypnoea and hypoxaemia, with few or no physical signs in the chest.

Although opportunistic infection was at first suspected, Mr Pottinger was in fact at an early stage in his treatment, at no time had he been seriously leucopenic and, despite his marked dyspnoea, he appeared clinically well. Fever suggests infection but is also seen as a manifestation of drug toxicity. In fact further investigation, including serial viral titres and microbiological examination of bronchoalveolar lavage fluid and transbronchial lung biopsies, failed to reveal an infective aetiology and specifically no evidence of *Pneumocystis carinii* infection. The histological picture was non-specific with an alveolar and interstitial infiltrate of mixed inflammatory cells. A therapeutic trial of high-dose co-trimoxazole was without benefit but sustained clinical and radiographic improvement followed treatment with corticosteroids and idiosyncratic bleomycin toxicity was accepted as the probable cause.

Pulmonary toxicity associated with bleomycin occurs in about 3–4% of treated patients. It is a dose-related phenomenon with a marked increase in risk when the cumulative doses exceeds 400 mg. This side effect can be unpredictable, however, and fatal pulmonary bleomycin toxicity has been reported at a much lower cumulative dose ($\sim$ 100 mg). The risk is increased in association with advanced age (over 70 years), previous radiotherapy, pre-existing pulmonary impairment and renal insufficiency. Two apparently distinct presentations are seen. The first and most common picture consists of interstitial pneumonitis which progresses to fibrosis. A hypersensitivity pneumonitis is also seen. Patients in both groups will respond to corticosteroids, but long-term therapy is usually required and withdrawal of steroids may lead to recurrence. In severe cases associated with marked dyspnoea, hypoxaemia and prominent radiographic abnormalities the overall mortality is about 50%.

Many cytostatic drugs have shown potential pulmonary toxicity (Cooper *et al.* 1986), bleomycin, busulphan and methotrexate being by far the most commonly implicated drugs. Among those included in Mr Pottinger's regimen procarbazine and vinblastine have also been associated with pneumonitis. The former is a rare cause of a hypersensitivity pneumonitis, characterized by fever, skin rash and peripheral blood eosinophilia. Pulmonary toxicity associated with vinblastine is less well documented and has only been reported when used in combination with mitomycin C.

Further reading

COOPER, J. A. D., WHITE, D. A. and MATTHAY, R. A. (1986) Drug-induced pulmonary disease. *American Review of Respiratory Disease,* **133,** 321.

RIES, F., SCULIER, J. P. and KLASTERSKY, J. (1987) Diffuse bilateral pneumopathies in patients with cancer. *Cancer treatment Reviews,* **14,** 119.

Case 30

Answers

1. There is a large area of consolidation with an air-fluid level in the left middle and lower zones.
2. The radiographic abnormality and Mrs Reeves' clinical deterioration were the result of a pyogenic lung abscess.

A lung abscess results when pulmonary infection by pyogenic organisms gives rise to parenchymal necrosis and cavitation. The clinical differential diagnosis of cavitating pulmonary lesions was considered in Answer 2. However, in a febrile postoperative patient with no prior history of respiratory symptoms and a normal preoperative chest film the diagnosis of lung abscess should present no difficulty. Typically symptoms have an onset over 24–48 hours with malaise, fever and chills (or even rigors). These symptoms are accompanied by cough and chest pain which is frequently pleuritic but which may also be poorly localized and aching in character. Drainage of the abscess contents via the bronchial tree results in the production of copious amounts of purulent sputum which is often bloodstained. Life-threatening haemoptysis may occur. Foul-smelling sputum is strongly suggestive of anaerobic infection. Rupture of the abscess into the pleural cavity results in an empyema or pyopneumothorax.

Physical signs over a lung abscess are often limited to a dull percussion note with reduction in breath sounds and transient pleural friction. Classical 'amphoric' breath sounds are seldom elicited. Finger clubbing is a late feature but may develop over a period of weeks, especially when drainage of the abscess cavity is inadequate. There is almost invariably a marked peripheral blood leucocytosis. The microbiological cause is usually established from aerobic and anaerobic cultures of sputum and blood.

Lung abscesses may arise in a number of ways (Table A30.1) and a wide variety of micro-organisms may be implicated. By far the commonest cause is 'aspiration' of infected material from within the respiratory tract when a mixed bacterial population (aerobic and anaerobic streptococci, fusiform bacilli, spirochaetes, staphylococci and pneumococci) is encountered. Although Mrs Reeves had suffered a lower limb deep venous thrombosis, there was nothing to suggest an embolic event prior to her clinical deterioration and secondary infection of pulmonary infarcts is a rare occurrence. Basal pneumonia and lung abscess may complicate sub-diaphragmatic infection (see Answer 3) following abdominal surgery, but there is nothing to suggest intra-abdominal infection in the case of Mrs Reeves and her lung abscess was not closely related to the diaphragm.

Lung abscesses secondary to pyaemia and septic venous embolism are closely related phenomena. In pyaemia venous blood is infected from septic thrombi in capillaries and small venules; similar lesions occurring in larger veins produce septic emboli.

Table A30.1 Mechanisms of lung abscess formation

A lung abscess may complicate:
Infection arising in the respiratory tract – 'aspiration abscesses' due to:
    Pre-existing respiratory infection, e.g. sinusitis, bronchiectasis
    Compromised integrity of the lower respiratory tract, e.g. impaired level of
        consciousness (anaesthesia, alcholic stupor, epilepsy); ineffective cough in
        postoperative, elderly or debilitated patients; achalasia; bulbar palsy
    Bronchial obstruction, e.g. by foreign body, bronchial carcinoma
Pneumonic consolidation
Blood-borne infection (pyaemic abscess, septic emboli)
Pulmonary infarction ('septic' infarct)
Chest trauma, e.g. penetrating chest wound or closed chest injury with subsequent
    infection of a haematoma via the respiratory passages
Subdiaphragmatic infection, e.g. subphrenic abscess, amoebic liver abscess

Both conditions tend to produce multiple, peripherally situated abscesses in which staphylococci and gram-negative bacteria are the usual pathogens and intravenous drug abusers the most commonly affected group. Rarely, embolic lung abscesses may result from bacterial endocarditis when an infected patent ductus arteriosus releases septic fragments into the pulmonary circulation.

Abscess formation is an occasional complication of pneumonic consolidation. It is an unusual feature of pneumococcal infection and occurs much more frequently in association with pneumonia due to Staphylococcus aureus and Klebsiella pneumoniae. Not all cavities represent abscesses, however. Thin-walled cysts (with or without an air-fluid level) may develop rapidly within an area of consolidation due to a check valve obstruction rather than actual lung necrosis. Such 'pneumatocoeles' are a particularly characteristic feature of staphylococcal pneumonia in infants. They may enlarge rapidly and frequently rupture into the pleural cavity with a resulting pneumothorax or pyopneumothorax.

Successful management is dependent upon adequate drainage of the abscess combined with appropriate antibiotic therapy. The latter will be determined by the nature of the infecting organism(s) and bacteriological sensitivity tests. In general terms, however, benzylpenicillin is the drug of choice for anaerobic pleuropulmonary infections. Mechanical drainage can usually be achieved by physiotherapy and posturing as determined by the anatomical location of the abscess. The lateral chest X-ray is usually sufficient for this purpose; bronchoscopy may also be of diagnostic value (localization of abscess, exclusion of bronchial obstruction) as well as having a useful therapeutic role. Foreign body bronchial obstruction producing distal suppuration requires bronchoscopic extraction which is best carried out with a rigid (rather than flexible) scope under general anaesthesia. This provides superior suction and better control over the airway – essential requirements if, as is sometimes the case, removal of the foreign body is followed by egress of much purulent material with the risk of flooding the bronchial tree.

Lung abscess secondary to a proximal obstructing bronchial neoplasm should be treated surgically provided that there are no contraindications to thoracotomy. Surgery may also be required for the treatment of an empyema. Rarely, lobectomy may be necessary if medical treatment fails or if, after bacteriological cure, residual localized bronchiectasis gives rise to significant symptoms uncontrollable by medical therapy.

Case 31

Answers

1. Barogenic rupture of the oesophagus.
2. Contrast radiographic examination of the oesophagus (e.g. dionosil or barium swallow).

The diagnosis of oesophageal rupture seldom poses any difficulty when there is a clear history of severe chest pain following an obvious predisposing event. The most common cause is iatrogenic when the various causes include oesophageal dilatation, the diagnostic use of flexible endoscopes and the therapeutic use of endo-oesophageal tubes (e.g. Celestin, Sengstaken–Blakemore tubes). Among the non-iatrogenic causes barogenic rupture may complicate the act of vomiting (Boerhaave's syndrome) but is also recognized in association with childbirth, defaecation, lifting heavy objects and, rarely, following the accidental discharge of compressed air into the oesophagus. Other rare causes include oesophageal carcinoma and external trauma.

In the case of Boerhaave's syndrome oesophageal rupture results from an acute rise intra-oesophageal pressure (with the

oesophagus functionally closed at both ends – by the cricopharyn-
geus and at the gastro-oesophageal junction) when vomiting and
the associated rise in intra-abdominal pressure occurs against a
closed glottis. A similar mechanism is believed to be responsible
for the mucosal tear of the Mallory–Weiss syndrome; this is
normally complicated only by haemorrhage but it can be the first
stage in a two-stage process that ends in a complete rupture. The
lesion is always in the distal oesophagus, usually on the left side
just above the gastro-oesophageal junction where the muscle layer
is deficient relative to the upper oesophagus and there is less
extra-mural support from adjacent mediastinal structures.

Mr Jamieson was unable to give a clear history, but the
circumstances surrounding his admission to hospital should have
resulted in a high level of suspicion from the outset. Pain is almost
invariable and has an abrupt onset in about 30% of patients. The
clinical presentation depends upon the site of the perforation.
Cervical perforations (usually iatrogenic) are commonly associated with subcutaneous emphysema, neck and substernal pain.
Upper back and abdominal pain are more usual with thoracic
perforations and acute cardiovascular (myocardial infarction,
dissecting aortic aneurysm) and upper abdominal emergencies
(perforated peptic ulcer, acute pancreatitis) enter the differential
diagnosis, particularly when the onset of pain is subacute and
follows the causal event only after some delay. Vomiting always
precedes the pain of oesophageal rupture whereas the converse is
true of myocardial infarction. Cough, dyspnoea, cyanosis, fever
and peripheral blood leucocytosis all occur commonly. Sternal
tenderness may be elicited and difficulty experienced when
passing a nasogastric tube.

The diagnosis is usually straightforward when typical symptoms
arise in an appropriate clinical setting. In Mr Jamieson's case the
absence of abdominal signs, normal abdominal films and normal
serum amylase level were strong pointers against an intra-
abdominal emergency and the initial chest radiograph was fully
consistent with oesophageal perforation. The plain chest film can
be expected to show features suggestive of perforation in about
90% of cases. A small, usually left-sided, pleural effusion is a
common early finding and this is often followed by the
development of a hydro- or pyo-pneumothorax as in the present
case. Other possible radiographic features include subcutaneous
emphysma, mediastinal widening, mediastinal air-fluid levels or a
pneumomediastinum. Confirmation of the diagnosis is by means of
contrast radiographic examination of the oesophagus which shows

the site of the perforation and demonstrates whether the leak is confined to the mediastinum or is free into the pleural cavity. Extravasation may be manifested by:

1. Free spillage of contrast into the pleural cavity.
2. A pseudodiverticulum caused by a localized cervical leak.
3. A narrow tract of contrast parallel and posterior to the oesophagus due to a mucosal laceration.

Non-operative treatment (nasogastric suction, parenteral nutrition and intensive antibiotic therapy) may be appropriate if the perforation is well drained back into the oesophageal lumen or when the patient is well with minimal symptomatology and no clinical evidence of sepsis. Absolute indications for surgical treatment include pneumothorax, pneumomediastinum, shock, systemic sepsis and respiratory failure. The procedure of choice for the distal oesophageal tears of Boerhaave's syndrome is primary surgical repair, but surgical management might also involve drainage alone, oesophageal exclusion and oesophagectomy. Early diagnosis is vital to the success of operative treatment. Significant delay is associated with progressive soiling of the mediastinum, local and systemic sepsis and greatly increased mortality. Primary closure may still be attempted if the tear is 4–6 hours old provided that mediastinal contamination is minimal. With greater delays, and when there is extensive mediastinal infection, treatment requires some form of oesophageal exclusion, intensive antibiotic therapy, adequate pleural drainage and intensive feeding (either intravenously or enterally via a gastrostomy or jejunostomy).

Case 32

Answers

1. The clinical picture is not that of classical polyarteritis nodosa, but the combined features strongly suggest a systemic vasculitis.
2. Prominent renal and pulmonary involvement in the disease process suggests either organ as a source of positive diagnostic

material. Transbronchial lung biopsies confirmed a necrotizing small vessel vasculitis – 'microscopic polyarteritis'.

3. Induction therapy should consist of cyclophosphamide combined with high dose prednisolone (see below).

Mr Williamson's illness bears a close resemblance to that described in the patient, Mr Petersen (Case 7), with Goodpasture's syndrome. There are the same features of glomerulitis and renal impairment (much less marked in the case of Mr Williamson) as well as changes consistent with pulmonary haemorrhage (a chest X-ray showing diffuse alveolar consolidation and a raised K_{co} (see Answer 7). However, joint symptoms – a prominent presenting feature in this case – and purpuric skin lesions are not found in Goodpasture's syndrome and their presence should suggest a systemic vasculitis.

Necrotizing vasculitis produces a wide spectrum of clinical and pathological features. Among those disorders affecting small and medium sized vessels clinical syndromes overlap to a significant degree, their pathogenesis is poorly understood and disease classifications use varying diagnostic criteria. Nevertheless, despite the confusion that surrounds this group of disorders, a number of fairly well defined clinical syndromes may be recognized: the major representatives are polyarteritis nodosa, allergic angiitis and granulomatosis ('Churg–Strauss vasculitis'), Wegener's granulomatosis and 'microscopic polyarteritis' – the differential diagnosis in the case of Mr Williamson. Rarely, alveolar haemorrhage complicates the 'immune complex vasculitis' of systemic lupus erythematosus (SLE), but a negative ANF virtually excludes this diagnosis, especially in a male subject. There is also no history of penicillamine ingestion – a rare cause of immune complex pulmonary vasculitis and glomerulonephritis.

Polyarteritis nodosa classically affects medium sized muscular arteries with angiographically demonstrable aneurysm formation affecting renal, mesenteric or hepatic vessels. Hypertension is common, particularly in relation to healed arteritis, and renal involvement is characterized by fibrinoid necrosis of the larger vessels and areas of infarction and ischaemia as the major abnormalities. Peripheral nervous system involvement is common and death is most commonly related to the severity of gut or renal disease. By contrast, lung involvement is rare in classical polyarteritis. However, a subgroup of patients may be recognized in whom vasculitis predominantly affects small vessels and is characterized by a necrotizing glomerulitis (with epithelial crescents) and interstitial nephritis but without macroscopic aneurysm formation. Such patients, with 'microscopic polyarteritis', appear to form a separate category (Savage *et al.*, 1985). A majority present (76%) with constitutional symptoms, with fever in 41% of patients and haemoptysis in about 30%, most of whom will show radiographic or functional evidence of intrapulmonary haemorrhage. Peripheral nervous system lesions are uncommon but all patients show anaemia, raised ESR and renal involvement with negative tests for hepatitis B surface antigen – features suggesting that microscopic polyarteritis is a separate entity, distinct from classical polyarteritis.

Wegener's granulomatosis is a rare disorder the cardinal features of which are a small vessel vasculitis with necrotizing granulomatous lesions in the upper and lower respiratory tract and an associated glomerulonephritis. Typically, patients present with a history of nasal discharge (22%) or sinusitis (67%) and, ultimately, the destructive granulomatous process may result in the classical saddle nose deformity. Pulmonary involvement most characteristically takes the form of multiple cavitating nodules (1–10 cm diameter). Other radiographic features include areas of segmental consolidation due to pulmonary infarction, occasional small pleural effusions, evidence of secondary infection and alveolar haemorrhage. The prognosis is most closely related to the presence and severity of renal involvement; over 70% of cases show abnormal renal biopsies at presentation, yet hypertension – in contrast to polyarteritis nodosa – is relatively uncommon. Anaemia, a markedly raised ESR and peripheral blood leucocytosis are the rule.

The Churg–Strauss syndrome describes a necrotizing granulomatous vasculitis which, like classical polyarteritis, affects medium sized vessels but which is strongly associated with allergic disorders and eosinophilia. A previous history of allergic rhinitis is common. Asthmatic symptoms are invariable and may precede other disease manifestations by months or even years. Active vasculitis is associated with fever, weight loss, anaemia, raised ESR and peripheral blood eosinophilia. Pulmonary infiltrates (40%), cardiovascular (40%) and neurological involvement (60%) all occur commonly although renal disease tends to be minor and progressive renal failure is rare.

The diagnosis of these disorders depends upon the demonstration of histological changes of vasculitis in affected organs. The appearances are usually non-specific, but when placed in the clinical context, the overall picture will often suggest the likely course of the disease and help to direct specific treatment. The recent demonstration of cytoplasmic anti-neutrophil (IgG) antibodies in Wegener's granulomatosis and microscopic polyarteritis is of uncertain pathogenetic and diagnostic significance, but the finding offers the promise of providing a useful marker of disease activity. Untreated systemic vasculitis has a poor prognosis with a five year survival of less than 15%. Therapy with corticosteroids, with or without an immunosuppressant, has transformed the outlook for most patients. The routine use of cytotoxic therapy appears to add nothing to the results of corticosteroid therapy in classical polyarteritis. For patients with Wegener's granulomatosis and microscopic polyarteritis the response to high dose steroids is improved by the addition of cyclophosphamide and this combined regime is the treatment of choice.

Reference and further reading

SAVAGE, C. O. S., WINEARLS, C. G., EVANS, D.G. *et al.* (1985) Microscopic polyarteritis: presentation, pathology, prognosis. *Quarterly Journal of Medicine*, **56,** 467.
SAWICKA, E. H. (1987) The necrotizing vasculitides. *Thorax*, **42,** 913.

Case 33

Answers

1. The second X-ray shows bilateral 'miliary' shadowing.
2. Miliary tuberculosis.

A range of diseases can produce a diffuse radiographic infiltrate and in clinical respiratory medicine one is not uncommonly faced with this wide differential diagnosis. Table A33.1 is not an exhaustive list of all of the possible causes but it provides a practical classification, based primarily upon the predominant pathological abnormality in the lung and it provides a framework into which most disorders can be fitted. In many cases of diffuse lung disease the definitive diagnosis will depend upon lung biopsy. However, the history, physical signs, the specific radiographic features and the results of less invasive investigations will often enable an accurate clinical diagnosis.

Table A33.1 Causes of lung disease associated with diffuse, bilateral radiographic shadowing

Intra-alveolar/Interstitial exudates
Non-inflammatory
    Pulmonary oedema
    Alveolar proteinosis
    Pulmonary haemorrhage, e.g. Goodpasture's syndrome, haemosiderosis
    Alveolar microlithiasis
Inflammatory
    Viral, 'atypical' pneumonia
    Non-infective 'inhalation' pneumonitis,
      e.g. lipoid pneumonia, Mendelson's syndrome
    Cryptogenic fibrosing alveolitis
    Drug-induced pneumonitis/fibrosis,
      e.g. due to bleomycin, busulphan, methotrexate

Granulomatous lung disorders
Sarcoidosis
Tuberculosis, histoplasmosis
Extrinsic allergic alveolitis
Berylliosis

Malignant infiltration
Lymphangitis carcinomatosa
Lymphproliferative disorders
Blood-borne metastases

Pulmonary dysplastic disorders
Histiocytosis-X
Tuberous sclerosis
Lympangioleiomyomatosis
Neurofibromatosis

Pneumoconioses secondary to inorganic dusts
Non-fibrogenic,
  e.g. stannosis, siderosis
Fibrogenic,
  e.g. silicosis, asbestosis, coal-worker's pneumoconiosis

Important features of the clinical history include the nature of the respiratory symptoms, their duration and the order in which they appeared and progressed. A careful occupational (work and leisure) history is essential, detailing any exposure to noxious fumes, gases, organic or inorganic dusts. Diagnostic clues may also be found in associated systemic symptoms, e.g. weight loss, haematuria, joint involvement. Particular note should be made of the presence or absence of pyrexia, finger clubbing (common in fibrosing alveolitis, bronchiectasis, asbestosis, alveolar proteinosis – unusual in tuberculosis, lymphangitis) and lung crackles. Granulomatous lung disorders, particularly sarcoidosis but also allergic alveolitis and miliary tuberculosis, tend to show relatively few chest signs in the acute stages. This contrasts with many of the interstitial lung disorders where crackles are more commonly found at all stages of the disease.

Occasionally the radiographic features may be highly specific and allow a precise diagnosis (e.g. alveolar microlithiasis). More often the appearances – the size and shape of individual shadows, their density and distribution – are relatively non-specific, but certain associated features (e.g. bilateral hilar gland enlargement suggesting sarcoidosis, pleural thickening/calcification suggesting asbestosis, rib destruction suggesting metastatic tumour) will often point to a particular cause.

The X-ray appearance alone may be sufficient to suggest tuberculosis when there is classic 'miliary mottling': fine (< 2 mm diameter), discrete shadows evenly distributed throughout the lungs from apex to base. However, variations on this classical description are common. Typically, the patient is febrile and ill with a history of weight loss, but these systemic features may be masked in patients taking corticosteroids, e.g. renal transplant recipients. In endemic regions, histoplasmosis and coccidioidomycosis will produce similar clinical and radiographic features. In the UK the differential diagnosis of the febrile patient with miliary shadows on the chest X-ray is even more limited: acute or subacute allergic alveolitis or, more commonly, bronchopneumonia (with lobular consolidation) being the other likely causes. Sarcoidosis may also enter the differential diagnosis, although patients with purely pulmonary sarcoid are seldom febrile.

As in the case of Mrs Harrison, there may be radiographic evidence of a healed primary tuberculous complex or postprimary lesion, providing an important clue to the diagnosis. The white cell count is usually normal as it was here, sometimes with a leucopenia or a relative lymphocytosis, and is of little value in the differential diagnosis. Hepatomegaly and splenomegaly are common features of miliary tuberculosis in children, but are unusual in adults. A careful search is justified for choroidal tubercles which are virtually pathognomonic, but these are present in only about 15% of cases in adults. The tuberculin test is usually positive but is of no real diagnostic value. It cannot be over-emphasized that the diagnosis is primarily a clinical one and when there is strong suspicion treatment must not await bacteriological confirmation. Direct sputum examination is usually negative and, in the past, this has contributed to diagnostic delay. Liver and bone marrow provide a source of positive diagnostic material in about one third of patients. However, the most useful examination in sputum negative miliary TB is fibreoptic bronchoscopy which permits a positive bacteriological diagnosis in over 80% of patients with minimal delay (Willcox *et al.* 1986).

Miliary tuberculosis is no longer a common disease and its pattern has changed. Formerly, this was classically a complication of primary childhood infection. Nowadays, it is seen mainly among elderly patients where it often takes a cryptic from ('cryptic disseminated tuberculosis') when the patient presents with an obscure fever and weight loss but with a normal chest X-ray. Because of its relative rarity and frequently atypical presentation there is a real danger that the diagnosis is not considered with the tragic result that a potentially curable disease is diagnosed only at autopsy. The index of suspicion therefore must be high, especially among susceptible groups, i.e. the elderly, those with immunosuppressive diseases (e.g. AIDS, Hodgkin's disease, hepatic cirrhosis), patients on long term corticosteroids or other immunosuppressant medication (e.g. transplant recipients), immigrants, diabetics, previous gastrectomy patients, drug addicts, alcoholics and 'down-and-outs'.

When Mrs Harrison first presented with an exacerbation of asthma she was found to have extensive radiographic changes suggesting previous tuberculosis; bacteriological findings were negative in keeping with inactive disease. For patients who have received an adequate period of treatment with effective antituberculous chemotherapy the risk of subsequent relapse is very low and long term follow-up is not necessary. Those who have been given inadequate treatment and patients who have complied poorly with previous treatment remain at risk and observation (for at least two years) could be justified. This increased risk of relapse also applies to patients like Mrs Harrison who have never received any chemotherapy. Treatment policies for such patients vary from centre to centre, from indefinite observation (with treatment when relapse occurs) to full antituberculous therapy 'as an insurance'.

In general, the greater the radiographic extent of the lesion, the greater the risk of subsequent relapse. A strong case could therefore have been made for giving Mrs Harrison antituberculous treatment when she was first seen, especially when it seemed likely that she would be exposed to further immunosuppressant therapy (corticosteroids) for her bronchial asthma.

Reference

WILLCOX, P. A., POTGEITER, P. D., BATEMAN, E. D. and BENATAR, S. R. (1986) Rapid diagnosis of sputum negative miliary tuberculosis using the flexible fibreoptic bronchoscope. *Thorax,* **41,** 681.

Case 34

Answers

1. There is no evidence of asbestos related disease.
2. There is evidence of chronic obstructive lung disease as well as clinical features strongly suggestive of obstructive sleep apnoea.
3. The defintive diagnosis of sleep apnoea syndrome requires a detailed polysomnographic study. There is controversy as to the number of physiological variables that should form the basis of a 'sleep study' in a suspected case. A conventional study includes a recording of the electroencephalogram (EEG), electro-oculogram (EOG) and electromyogram (EMG), permitting an analysis of sleep quality and sleep stage. Nasal and oral airflow are monitored to identify periods of apnoea and thoraco-abdominal motion is measured in order to distinguish central and obstructive sleep apnoeas. Finally, heart rate, ECG and arterial oxygen saturation (by ear oximetry) are monitored in order to assess the physiological consequences of apnoea and their severity.

It would seem likely that Mr Masters' breathlessness relates to a combination of chronic obstructive lung disease and obesity. There is no clinical, radiographic or physiological evidence of asbestos-related pulmonary or pleural disease. These parameters are insensitive indicators of early asbestosis but the relatively short duration of Mr Masters' asbestos exposure and its indirect nature suggests that he was an unlikely candidate for asbestosis which is generally associated with prolonged or intense asbestos exposure. Bi-basal lung crackles are an important, but non-specific, feature of asbestosis. However, their timing in the respiratory cycle (early inspiratory) suggests that in Mr Masters' case thay are a manifestation of his airways disease. Asbestosis, like other causes of diffuse pulmonary fibrosis, produces bi-basal crackles that are characteristically high-pitched, posture-dependent (diminish on leaning forwards) and late inspiratory in timing.

In addition to obstructive lung disease systematic enquiry revealed additional features of obstructive sleep apnoea. The importance of this and other sleep-related respiratory disorders has only begun to be appreciated over the last decade. Their significance in relation to a wide range of cardiopulmonary problems is beyond doubt and, with the advent of successful therapy, patients with suggestive clinical features warrant thorough investigation as outlined above.

Apnoea may be seen in normal individuals during sleep onset and during periods of rapid-eye-movement sleep. Such apnoeic episodes are brief (less than 15 seconds) and non-repetitive with a maximal frequency of about 12 apnoeas per hour of sleep. By contrast, the patient with clinically obvious sleep apnoea will have repetitive apnoeas which last longer than 15 seconds and are associated with reductions in arterial oxygen saturation. Sleep apnoea is classified as central, obstructive or mixed, depending upon the presence or absence of respiratory efforts: central apnoea is the result of failure to generate respiratory effort and is characterized by absence of chest wall movement; obstructive apnoea is caused by failure of the mechanisms responsible for maintaining airway patency during sleep – gas flow ceases due to occlusion of the upper airway but respiratory effort and chest wall movement persists. Pure central apnoea is rare and most adults with sleep apnoea show an obstructive or mixed pattern of abnormality.

The clinical symptoms of obstructive sleep apnoea may be subtle and the condition often goes unrecognized for long periods. The syndrome has been recognized in association acromegaly, hypothyroidism, mucopolysaccharidoses, micrognathia, tonsillar and adenoidal hypertrophy (the most common cause in children), all of which are associated with narrowing of the upper airway. Table A34.1 lists the major clinical features in adults. A history of loud snoring and excessive daytime sleepiness are usually present although the patient himself is commonly unaware of symptoms and it is important that a history is taken from family members. Obesity is noted in about 60% of patients and recent weight gain often precedes the onset of apnoeas. Snoring, a symptom of incomplete upper airway obstruction, often precedes other symptoms by some years. With the onset of apnoeas snoring becomes intermittent when it is interrupted by periods of silence and the patient is seen to make vigorous respiratory efforts. Each apnoeic episode is terminated by an arousal so that sleep is repeatedly disturbed. The patient may awake frequently and complain of insomnia. More often the patient claims to sleep well but complains that he feels unrefreshed by sleep.

The severity of the condition is extremely variable. About 10–15% of patients (those with the most severe nocturnal hypoxaemia) develop sustained pulmonary hypertension due to hypoxic pulmonary vasoconstriction, leading to right heart failure. Systemic hypertension is seen in about 60% of patients; although obesity is a contributory cause hypertension is also a feature in non-obese patients with sleep apnoea and the mechanism remains unclear.

Table A34.1   Clinical features of obstructive sleep apnoea

Symptoms	Signs
Loud snoring	Obesity
Unrefreshing sleep	Systemic hypertension
Abnormal motor activity in sleep	Pulmonary hypertension
Excessive daytime sleepiness	Polycythaemia
Personality changes	Right heart failure
Intellectual deterioration	Cardiac arrythmias
Morning headaches	
Hallucinations	
Sudden death?	

A variety of cardiac arrythmias may be seen in association with apnoeas and this has led to the suggestion that the syndrome may be responsible for sudden death during sleep. The most common arrythmia is a moderate bradycardia (30–50 beats/min) during apnoeas. In a small proportion of patients more significant abnormalities (profound bradycardia, ventricular extrasystoles and runs of ventricular tachycardia) are seen.

Patients with severe disease (as determined by the severity arterial oxygen desaturation during sleep) undoubtedly warrant treatment. However, little is known of the natural history of mild or moderate sleep apnoea and it is unclear as to whether or not treatment is necessary for these groups. Any predisposing causes (e.g. hypothyroidism, adenoidal/tonsillar hypertrophy) should be identified and treated. Simple treatment measures such as avoidance of respiratory depressants (alcohol and sedatives) may suffice in some patients. Most obese patients will show significant symptomatic and objective improvement with weight reduction and some patients respond dramatically. More specific therapy is frequently required however.

The available treatments include drug therapy, surgery and nasal continuous positive airways pressure. The most effective drug is protryptiline which increases the tone of upper airway muscles, but its value is limited by side effects and its efficacy, both in the short and long term, is open to doubt. Uvulopalatopharyngoplasty has been popularized as an effective surgical means of increasing the size of the oropharyngeal lumen; short term improvement is seen in roughly 50% of patients but once again long term efficacy is unproven. Tracheostomy bypasses the site of upper airway obstruction and provides immediate and effective control of symptoms. The operation has been all but supplanted, however, by the application of a continuous positive pressure to the airway via a tightly fitting nasal mask (nasal CPAP). A positive pressure in the upper airway throughout the respiratory cycle acts as a pneumatic splint and effectively prevents upper airway obstruction. It is generally well tolerated and, in most centres, has now become the treatment of choice for obstructive sleep apnoea.

Further reading

STRADLING, J. R. and PHILLIPSON, E. A. (1986) Breathing disorders during sleep. *Quarterly Journal of Medicine*, **58**, 3.

STROHL, K. P., CHERNIACK, N. S. and GOTHE, B. (1986) Physiologic basis of therapy for sleep apnoea. *American Review of Respiratory Disease*, **134**, 791.

Case 35

Answers

1. Allergic bronchopulmonary aspergillosis.
2. Treatment with systemic steroids will suppress the associated inflammatory response in the bronchial wall and vigorous chest physiotherapy will usually lead to re-expansion of the collapsed lobe. Occasionally, this fails and bronchoscopy is required with suction of the tenacious mucus plugs.

The correct diagnosis is suggested by the patient's previous history which is in keeping with bronchial asthma, her peripheral blood eosinophilia (eosinophil count $> 0.55 \times 10^9/l$) and the combination of radiographic abnormalities, i.e. lobar collapse associated with non-segmental shadowing, corresponding to an area of eosinophilic consolidation, in the contralateral lung. While allergic bronchopulmonary aspergillosis (ABPA) occasionally complicates the course of late onset, skin test negative, 'intrinsic' asthma, it is much more strongly associated with the atopic state and Mrs Eastcliffe's history of atopic eczema and rhinitis and her strong family history of asthma are fully consistent with this clinical diagnosis.

Allergic bronchopulmonary aspergillosis is recognized in about 8% of all patients with bronchial asthma and, in the UK, it accounts for about 80% of all cases of asthmatic pulmonary eosinophilia. Its manifestations relate not to any primary effect of the fungus , but to an altered host response – mediated by specific antibodies – in patients who have become sensitized to aspergillus antigens. The main diagnostic features are: a history of asthma, recurrent radiographic shadowing, peripheral blood eosinophilia (usually modest, e.g. $0.6–1.5 \times 10^9/l$), and a positive immediate skin prick test to *Aspergillus fumigatus* antigen. The majority of affected patients will also show a delayed positive (Arthus type) skin test reaction, positive serum precipitins to *Aspergillus fumigatus* and positive sputum cultures. These features are more variable however. The demonstration of serum precipitins is closely dependent upon laboratory technique and the fungus may be seen or grown from sputum only intermittently.

Even the major diagnostic criteria may be somewhat variable: asthmatic symptoms are not prominent in all patients and episodes of pulmonary eosinophilia are not always closely related to exacerbations of asthma. It is not unusual therefore to find that previous episodes of pulmonary infiltration have been mis-diagnosed as being due to pneumonia, as in the case of Mrs Eastcliffe, or even pulmonary tuberculosis. Diagnostic difficulty is greatest among non-atopic patients in whom asthmatic symptoms are inconspicuous or even absent and in whom the radiographic picture is one of lobar collapse or collapse of an entire lung in the absence of pulmonary infiltrates (Berkin *et al.*, 1982). In such circumstances bronchial carcinoma may be diagnosed in error, although the findings at bronchoscopy will readily differentiate. Mucus plugging due to this and other causes must be considered in the differential diagnosis of bronchial obstruction (Table A35.1).

There is no pathognomonic radiographic abnormality, but the constellation of changes seen in any individual patient over a period of time may be virtually diagnostic. Abnormal radiographic shadowing is of two main types. The first group of shadows results from pulmonary eosinophilic 'pneumonia' and typically these

Table A35.1 Causes of bronchial obstruction

Bronchial carcinoma
Mucus plugging
Inhaled foreign body
Extrinsic compression from hilar lymphadenopathy,
   e.g. primary tuberculosis
Tuberculous bronchostenosis (Brock's syndrome)
Bronchial adenoma
Other benign intrabronchial tumours
Intrabronchial metastases

consist of transient, non-segmental areas of homogeneous consolidation. They frequently show a perihilar distribution and predominantly affect the upper lobes. The second group of shadows represents manifestations of bronchial obstruction or dilatation and consists of various types of 'tubular' shadow. Band-like shadows are seen when secretions fill a dilated bronchus. These characteristically give way to parallel line or 'tram-line' shadows following the expectoration of purulent sputum plugs – a feature in about a third of patients – which may be responsible for recurrent episodes of pulmonary or lobar collapse as in the present case. Repeated episodes of pulmonary eosinophilia and the tissue damaging reactions, mediated by precipitating antibody, with which they are associated, lead to permanent radiographic abnormalities. Aerated but shrunken upper lobes may be seen similar to the extrinsic allergic alveolitis of bird fancier's lung. In other patients a particularly characteristic form of saccular bronchiectasis is seen which involves proximal bronchi.

In the majority of patients recurrent episodes of pulmonary eosinophilia result in progressive, insidious deterioration. Some workers have commented upon a burnt-out stage when episodes of pulmonary eosinophilia become less frequent or totally disappear, but compared to a control group of asthmatics matched for age, sex and duration of asthma, patients with ABPA show greater functional impairment and lower average values for FEV_1 and VC. They also tend to have less readily reversible airflow obstruction and often show impaired gas transfer to a degree which correlates with the extent of pulmonary fibrosis and other evidence of permanent lung damage.

The management of asthmatic symptoms is essentially the same whether a patient has ABPA or not, although patients with ABPA –

166

for the reasons given above – are likely to require more extensive treatment and a greater proportion will be steroid-dependent. In acute episodes of ABPA treatment with systemic steroids improves symptoms and also hastens the resolution of abnormal radiographic shadowing as well as re-aeration of a collapsed lobe. Some studies have suggested that long term treatment with steroids might prevent recurrent episodes of pulmonary eosinophilia, but this has not been confirmed in a controlled study. To date neither corticosteroids nor antifungal therapy has been shown convincingly to alter the natural history of the condition.

Reference and further reading

BERKIN, K. E., VERNON, D. R. H. and KERR, J. W. (1982) Lung collapse caused by allergic bronchopulmonary aspergillosis in non-asthmatic patients. *British Medical Journal*, **285**, 552.

McCARTHY, D. S. and PEPYS, J. (1971) Allergic bronchopulmonary aspergillosis. Clinical Immunology: (1) Clinical features. *Clinical Allergy*, **1**, 261.

Case 36

Answers

1. Small cell anaplastic carcinoma of the bronchus.
2. Confirmation of the diagnosis requires bronchoscopy and biopsy. Loss of definition of the right heart border reflects collapse or consolidation affecting the (right) middle lobe which was found, at bronchoscopy, to be occluded by obvious tumour tissue.
3. (a) The electrolyte abnormalities are probably the result of inappropriate antidiuretic hormone secretion.
   (b) The haematological abnormalties (thrombocytopenia, leuco-erythroblastic blood picture) strongly suggest metastatic bone marrow infiltration.

Small cell lung cancer is one of the four main histopathological types of bronchial carcinoma. Two subtypes are recognized: 'oat' cell tumours, where cells bear a morphological resemblance to small lymphocytes, and the 'intermediate' subtype which includes all other morphological variants. Together, as small cell lung cancer (SCLC), these account for about 20% of all malignant bronchial neoplasms. Quite apart from the individual pathological appearance of these tumours, there are significant clinical differences and major differences in terms of their biological behaviour – in comparison with other tumour types – that categorize SCLC as a distinct disease entity. They show a faster growth rate, they are more highly invasive and they show a greater potential for early and more widespread dissemination than is the case for 'non-small cell' tumours (squamous carcinoma, adenocarcinoma, large cell anaplastic carcinoma).

Nearly all patients with SCLC are symptomatic at the time of presentation and the duration of symptoms tends to be shorter than for other histologies, averaging three months. By contrast, the average duration of symptoms is around eight months for squamous cell tumours, whilst as many as a quarter of patients with adenocarcinomas may be asymptomatic at diagnosis. As with squamous cell carcinoma, the majority of small cell tumours (80–90%) arise 'centrally' in the bronchial tree and most patients present with symptoms related to the primary tumour: cough, dyspnoea, haemoptysis. By virtue of their greater invasive potential, however, rather more patients with SCLC than with other tumour types present with symptoms referrable to regional extension of disease: superior vena caval obstruction, recurrent laryngeal nerve palsy, phrenic nerve palsy, Horner's syndrome. Systemic metastases are present in as many as 80% of patients at diagnosis, with clear implications for management (see below).

Although there is no pathognomonic radiographic appearance, a central tumour mass with prominent hilar enlargement or mediastinal widening is particularly common (Figure A36.1); mediastinal involvement secondary to other cell types is rarely as apparent. Peripheral tumour masses or infiltrates which are most characteristic of adenocarcinoma are uncommon with SCLC and central cavitation, a feature of 10–20% of squamous carcinomas, is rare.

Among their distinctive biological characteristics is a well recognized propensity for producing a wide variety of peptide hormones including ACTH, ADH, calcitonin and serotonin. Of the related clinical syndromes only ectopic Cushing's syndrome and the syndrome of inappropriate antidiuretic hormone secretion (SIADH) occur at all commonly. The latter is characterized by a dilutional hyponatraemia with serum hyposmolality and continued

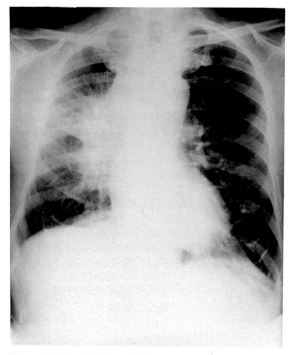

Figure A36.1 Small cell anaplastic carcinoma of the bronchus: mediastinal widening and grossly enlarged right hilum with radiating line shadows–'sunburst' appearance

renal sodium excretion with a less than maximally dilute urine; the diagnostic criteria also require normal renal and adrenal function and the absence of fluid volume depletion. A subclinical disorder of water balance (e.g. abnormal response to a water load) may occur in as many as 60% of SCLC patients at diagnosis, but clinically detectable SIADH is apparent in only about 8% of cases. Associated symtomatology (lethargy, confusion, drowsiness, nausea, irritability) is unusual unless hyponatraemia is severe – plasma sodium less than 120 mmol/l. More serious manifestations including fits, coma and focal neurological signs may occur, leading to clinical suspicion of CNS metastases (also a cause of SIADH), with plasma sodium levels below 110 mmol/l. The syndrome responds rapidly to effective treatment directed against the underlying disease. The biochemical abnormality improves with fluid restriction and certain forms of drug therapy (dimethyl-

169

chlortetracycline, lithium) which may be useful as adjunctive treatment whist awaiting a response to cytotoxic chemotherapy.

In the case of Mrs Graham, therefore, the combined clinical picture (short history, evidence of hepatic and bone marrow abnormality), radiological features (prominent mediastinal involvement) and biochemical evidence of SIADH should strongly suggest a diagnosis of SCLC, especially in a previously heavy smoker. The haematological abnormalities, hepatomegaly and mediastinal lymphadenopathy could also be explained on the basis of a malignant lymphoma (a rare cause of SIADH), but the absence of superficial lymphadenopathy and the radiographic evidence of middle lobe collapse, indicating an intrabronchial abnormality, render this less likely. A dilutional hyponatraemia may also be seen in patients with severe congestive cardiac failure. Mrs Graham's presenting symptoms, her history of hypertension and the presence of cardiomegaly, hepatomegaly and abnormal liver function could all be explained on this basis. This diagnosis would not however account for the abnormal blood picture or for all of the X-ray abnormalities.

Its potential for early and widespread dissemination severely limits the role of surgery in the management of SCLC. Surgery remains appropriate, however, for a small group of patients who, after detailed staging, are found to have stage I disease (tumour confined to the lung without evidence of regional lymphadenopathy). For the majority of patients with more widespread disease combination chemotherapy is the mainstay of treatment. A variety of regimens are capable of producing high tumour response rates (80–90%) with a small proportion of patients achieving long-term disease remission. However median survival is poor averaging 12–18 months depending upon the initial extent of disease. The majority of patients relapse and die within two years of diagnosis. Radiotherapy to the primary tumour probably improves local disease control but does not improve median survival in chemotherapy-treated patients and its precise role remains contentious.

Further reading

HAINSWORTH, J. D., WORKMAN, R. and GRECO, F. A. (1983) Management of the syndrome of inappropriate antidiuretic hormone secretion in small cell lung cancer. *Cancer*, **51**, 161.
HANSEN, H. H. (1987) Chemotherapy of small cell carcinoma: a review. *The Quarterly Journal of Medicine*, **63**, 275.

Case 37

Answers

1. Cystic fibrosis.
2. (a) A sweat test.
   (b) Estimation of faecal fat excretion.

The vast majority of patients with cystic fibrosis present and are diagnosed during infancy but a significant minority, 6% of all cases in one series (Penketh *et al.* 1987), are diagnosed during adult life. Few patients are newly diagnosed beyond the age of 30 and only a handful after 40 years of age. Nevertheless, it is clear that the natural history of the disease does vary and its slow rate of progression in some patients may lead to delayed diagnosis. The main clinical features are chronic bronchopulmonary infection, pancreatic insufficiency, a high sweat sodium concentration and a family history of cystic fibrosis. However, pancreatic insufficiency may be absent and a positive family history (even when this is available) is frequently not found. These considerations emphasize the need to consider the diagnosis in any patient with chronic or recurrent bronchopulmonary infection, especially if there is also evidence of malabsorption, when the sweat test should be included in the diagnostic work-up. In Mr Sissons' case the demonstration of steatorrhoea (faecal fat excretion, 12 g/24 h) confirmed pancreatic exocrine insufficiency and sweat sodium concentrations on two occasions of 90 and 94 mmol/l confirmed the diagnosis of cystic fibrosis.

Even in the absence of gastrointestinal symptoms, the pattern of bronchopulmonary involvement may be sufficient to suggest the diagnosis. Affected patients generally have a long history of respiratory infection dating from childhood. Clinical and radiographic signs of bronchiectasis are concentrated in the upper lobes and the sputum yields only a narrow spectrum of 'typical' pathogens. *Staphylococcus aureus* is generally the predominant organism early in the course of the disease. This is gradually supplanted by *Pseudomonas aeruginosa*, particularly 'mucoid' strains, and this organism is almost invariably present in the sputum of adult sufferers with established respiratory disease.

Obviously any one of the above features occurring in isolation has little diagnostic value and it is their association which should suggest cystic fibrosis. Bronchiectasis from other causes (Table

A37.1) not uncommonly has its origin during childhood. However, with the exception of postprimary tuberculosis, extrinsic allergic alveolitis and allergic bronchopulmonary aspergillosis (ABPA), the other causes of bronchiectasis produce either focal changes (e.g. foreign body, bronchial adenoma, primary tuberculosis) or more generalized respiratory involvement which tends to be concentrated in the lower rather than the upper lobes. Mr Sissons' early history of respiratory symptoms suggests the possibility of asthma and the radiographic abnormality is certainly consistent with ABPA but his non-atopic status and negative aspergillus precipitins virtually exclude this as a primary diagnosis. In fact *Aspergillus fumigatus* frequently colonizes the lung in cystic fibrosis and about half of the patients have positive skin reactions and about a quarter have serum precipitins to this fungus. ABPA and aspergilloma are both seen as rare complications.

Table A37.1 Causes of bronchiectasis

Congenital	*Acquired*
Congenital bronchiectasis:	*Children*
Bronchomalacia (Williams–Campbell syndrome)	Inhaled foreign body
	Primary tuberculosis
Pulmonary sequestration	Pneumonia
Unilateral emphysema (McLeod's syndrome)	Whooping cough
	Measles
'Immotile cilia syndrome' (e.g. Kartagener's syndrome)	*Adults*
Other cases of ciliary dysfunction (e.g. Young's syndrome)	Pneumonia
	Pulmonary tuberculosis
Congenital disorders pre-disposing to bronchiectasis	Allergic bronchopulmonary aspergillosis
Cystic fibrosis	Bronchial adenoma
Hypogammaglobulinaemia	Disorders producing extensive pulmonary fibrosis and disorganization of lung architecture
	Chagas' disease

In adults, as in children, pulmonary disease and respiratory infection in particular is by far the single most important cause of morbidity and mortality. Clinical deterioration is paralleled by progressive airflow obstruction. Right heart failure is a common terminal event but is relatively unusual during the course of the disease. Haemoptysis occurs at some stage in the majority of patients and spontaneous pneumothorax is a complication in about

20% of cases. Nasal polyposis and sinusitis are frequent upper airways manifestations.

Adults with cystic fibrosis tend to show a milder degree of malabsorption than is the case in children. Severe symptomatic steatorrhoea is unusual and about 10–15% of adolescents will have no symptoms of malabsorption at all. The correct use of pancreatic enzyme supplements improves nutritional status and provides effective control in symptomatic patients, making dietary restrictions unnecessary in the majority. Greater gastrointestinal morbidity in adults is associated with small bowel obstruction (meconium ileus equivalent), a complication in about 20% of cases. The syndrome is characterized by intermittent episodes of colicky abdominal pain, distension, constipation and palpable abdominal faecal masses. Most cases respond to conservative management with rehydration, oral and rectal administration of N-acetylcysteine, attention to diet and pancreatic enzyme replacement. Other gastrointestinal complications include rectal prolapse, intussusception, diabetes mellitus (10%), hepatomegaly and abnormal liver function tests (10%), portal hypertension (rare) and gallstones (rare).

Reference

PENKETH, A. R. L., WISE, A., MEARNS, M. B. *et al* (1987) Cystic fibrosis in adolescents and adults. *Thorax*, **42**, 526.

Case 38

Answers

1. Bronchial carcinoma.
2. Mrs Cox's clinical deterioration was due to cardiac tamponade. Postmortem examination confirmed pericardial and chest wall involvement by a primary bronchial neoplasm arising in the lingular segment of the left upper lobe.

Cough is almost an invariable symptom among patients with bronchial carcinoma because the subjects are usually smokers. However, the patient will often describe a recent change in the character of his cough (e.g. less productive than usual or more persistent). Weight loss of more than 6.5 kg is a presenting feature in 55% of patients. Chest pain is a common symptom and can be a feature of both centrally and peripherally located tumours. Central neoplasms may give rise to deep-seated, poorly localized discomfort related to invasion of mediastinal structures or to pleuritic pain secondary to pneumonia complicating bronchial obstruction. In the case of peripheral lesions chest pain may arise from direct invasion of the parietal pleura or chest wall. The continuous nature of Mrs Cox's pain is in keeping with chest wall involvement, but certain features – pain worse when lying flat, radiation to the shoulder and left arm – suggest pericardial pain.

Whereas breathlessness due to central tumours is secondary to bronchial obstruction, that due to peripheral neoplasms results from the 'space occupying' effect of the tumour. Dyspnoea due to a large pleural effusion may reflect direct pleural involvement from a peripheral neoplasm, pleural metastases (malignant effusions) or lymphatic obstruction associated with central mediastinal lymph node involvement (non-malignant effusion). In Mrs Cox's case increased breathlessness relates to the combined effect of the primary tumour and unilateral diaphragmatic paralysis due to phrenic nerve involvement. In an otherwise normal subject unilateral paralysis of the diaphragm is associated with an approximate 20% fall in ventilatory capacity and may produce no symptoms. Dyspnoea is more likely to result when phrenic nerve palsy complicates an underlying neoplasm in a patient whose lung function is already compromised by pre-existing chronic obstructive lung disease.

The overall clinical picture in a middle-aged smoker strongly suggests bronchial carcinoma. Although fibreoptic bronchoscopy yielded negative findings, in keeping with a peripheral neoplasm, the location of the primary tumour is suggested by the radiographic abnormality: the left heart border is normally clearly defined because it lies adjacent to the expanded lingular segment of the left upper lobe. When the lingula is abnormal (due to tumour, consolidation, collapse) it acquires the same ('soft tissue') density as the heart, the silhouette of which is then lost as was reported in Mrs Cox's initial chest film. The lingula is closely related to the pericardium overlying the left ventricle and also to the left phrenic nerve which, in the lower part of its intrathoracic course, passes in front of the left hilum to lie between the parietal pericardium (covering the left ventricle) and the mediastinal pleura. Regional spread of tumour from this primary site would readily account therefore for both the radiographic abnormality and the observed clinical manifestations of pericardial and phrenic nerve involvement.

Against this clinical background Mrs Cox's rapid deterioration, characterized by low blood pressure and cardiac output with elevation of jugular venous pressure and an increase in cardiac size (due to pericardial effusion), should suggest tamponade. In addition to faint heart sounds the other clinical features of tamponade include tachycardia, narrow pulse pressure, pulsus paradoxus (a fall in systolic blood pressure of 10 mmHg or more on inspiration) and a paradoxical rise in central venous pressure on inspiration (Kussmaul's sign). The ECG, chest X-ray and echocardiograph will provide confirmatory evidence of pericardial fluid and the latter may also suggest tamponade (e.g. when there is beat-to-beat pendular motion of the heart, collapse or 'buckling' of the right atrial wall on inspiration and obliteration of the right ventricular cavity in early diastole). However, the need for specific intervention (pericardiocentesis) and the haemodynamic significance of the effusion are most reliably determined from a careful clinical assessment. In the case of Mrs Cox repeated pericardial aspiration yielded heavily bloodstained fluid containing many malignant cells. This provided short term symptomatic relief but, despite pericardial instillation of cytotoxic therapy, long term control was unsuccessful and she soon succumbed.

Case 39

Answers

1. Occupational asthma due to barn dust.
2. An occupational aetiology may be diagnosed from characteristic changes in peak flow records maintained over periods at and away from work. Skin test reactions, detection of specific IgE serum antibodies and bronchial provocation testing may also play a useful diagnostic role (see below).

Occupational lung disease among farmers has been recognized since the eighteenth century when Ramazzini, the father of occupational medicine, described asthma in grain handlers. In the

1930s a form of extrinsic allergic alveolitis (farmer's lung) was recognized and more recently still, silo-filler's lung – a toxic pneumonitis related to the inhalation of nitrogen dioxide – has been described. Rarely, respiratory symptoms may follow the misuse of paraquat or through the inhalation of antifungal sprays. The breathless farm worker may therefore present a diagnostic challenge and it behoves the physician always to consider an occupational cause.

A careful history will usually reveal work-related symptoms, the character and timing of which will often suggest the specific cause. Silo-filler's lung is seen after acute exposure to nitrogen dioxide which is liberated from silage at an early stage in its fermentation. Cases occur sporadically, usually as a result of carelessness or poor education, when a farmer is exposed to the gas after entering a freshly filled and poorly ventilated tower silo. Because nitrogen dioxide is not particularly irritant the initial exposure often passes unnoticed, but within hours the farmer develops cough and breathlessness which may progress to pulmonary oedema. In some cases this acute response subsides only to be followed, some weeks later, by progressive dyspnoea due to obliterative bronchiolitis. Deaths have resulted during both stages of the disease. Treatment with corticosteroids may improve the prognosis and reduce pulmonary damage, but prevention is paramount and requires that farmers are educated in safe working practices.

Farmer's lung has become less common in recent years as farmers have changed from the use of hay to silage. The workforce is much better informed about the potential hazard and farmers are also more knowledgeable about prevention (e.g. correct methods of handling hay, use of protective headgear). Nevertheless, it remains an important problem, being seen in up to 5% of farm workers. The diagnosis is suggested by a history of fever, myalgia, dry cough and breathlessness developing 4–8 hours after exposure to stored mouldy hay. Recurrent exposure commonly results in malaise and weight loss. The characteristic clinical finding is that of inspiratory lung crackles, with radiographic pulmonary infiltration, a restrictive defect of ventilation and impaired gas transfer. The demonstration of serum precipitins to thermophilic actinomycetes provides confirmation. In practice, the clinical diagnosis is often less straightforward. In 'chronic' farmer's lung there may be no clear history of intermittent episodes of acute disease and serum precipitins are usually absent if exposure has not occurred for three or more years. At the same time, precipitins may be found in up to 20% of healthy, asymptomatic farm workers.

Some patients with farmer's lung also develop IgE antibodies to fungal spores and wheeze which is not normally a feature may then occur. Furthermore, fever and myalgia, although suggestive of alveolitis, may also be features of the late stage of some asthmatic reactions.

In the case of Mr Jessop the overall clinical picture points to a diagnosis of asthma, although some of the features are potentially misleading. His symptoms of rhinitis, conjunctivitis and associated breathlessness during the day suggests type I allergy which is characteristic of asthma but, as mentioned above, may also be a present in some patients with farmer's lung. Equally, his more severe breathlessness occurring later in the evenings would be consistent, in terms of its timing, with either allergic alveolitis or the late stage of a dual asthmatic reaction. However, the absence of lung crackles and of any abnormal radiographic shadowing point away from an alveolitis. The lung function abnormalities are also inconsistent with this explanation. A single set of lung function results may contribute little to the diagnosis of asthma which, by definition, requires demonstration of variability in airflow obstruction. In this instance, however, the results are helpful, being suggestive of asthma and quite unlike the results that would be expected in farmer's lung. Thus, the K_{co} is high (it is reduced in allergic alveolitis) and, in the presence of airflow limitation, asthma is the most likely cause for this; similar findings are seen with other causes of inspiratory obstruction. It is also worthy of note that the FEV_1 and FVC are reduced to a similar extent so that the FEV_1/FVC ratio is normal. This might appear to suggest restriction but the TLC is increased (the lungs are hyperinflated). The RV is also raised with an abnormally high RV/TLC ratio indicating air trapping, a typical feature of airflow obstruction. Simple spirometry will sometimes therefore give a misleading impression and fail to suggest an obstructive defect. In this case the acute response to bronchodilator (10% increase in FEV_1) is also less than that which one typically associates with asthma. This is not unusual, however, in association with severe asthma when the initial response to therapy often produces reductions in TLC and RV without, at first, any significant changes in FEV_1, FVC or peak flow. The antigen-induced late asthmatic response is considered to involve inflammatory changes rather than simple bronchoconstriction and limited responsiveness to bronchodilators is the rule. Mr Jessop himself had noted a poor response to inhaled salbutamol and therapy with corticosteroids was clearly indicated.

Occupational asthma is variable airway narrowing causally related to agents inhaled in the working environment. A large number of agents (well over 200) used at work have been implicated and with increased awareness of the problem and the introduction of new materials into industry the range of substances causing occupational asthma will increase. Its recognition is of obvious importance because avoidance of exposure to the causal agent may be followed by complete remission. In the UK affected patients are eligible for industrial compensation, but only in relation to a restricted list of seven sensitizing agents (platinum salts, isocyanates, epoxy resins, colophony, proteolytic enzymes, laboratory animals and flour and grain dust).

Occupational asthma may occur in up to 15% of farm workers. As with other causes of occupational asthma the diagnosis depends primarily upon a careful history although this approach clearly has its disadvantages particularly when compensation is involved. Self-recorded measurements of peak flow can be useful, but these require continued and uncontrolled work exposures which may not be appropriate in a patient with severe occupational asthma. They require a considerable commitment on the part of the doctor and the worker and their interpretation is often difficult. Positive skin tests or detection of specific IgE might help but the sensitivity and specificity of individual allergen extracts needs to be known. Bronchial provocation testing has only a small diagnostic role. It is time-consuming, requires careful attention to detail and can be dangerous. It may be justified for precise diagnosis when it may be necessary for the affected worker to leave the industry, or to determine the specific cause in a complex industrial environment, or when a previously unrecognized cause of occupational asthma is being investigated.

Further reading

BURGE, P. S. (1987) Problems in the diagnosis of occupational asthma. *British Journal of Diseases of the Chest*, **81**, 105.
CHAN-YEUNG, M. and LAM, S. (1986) Occupational asthma. *American Review of Respiratory Diseases*, **133**, 686.

Case 40

Answers

1. The area of shadowing situated anteriorly on the plain chest X-ray – in the cardiophrenic angle – is shown to be a heterogeneous mass displacing the heart posteriorly. The radiographic density is variable and indicates a mixed composition with areas of fat, air and soft tissue. The cross-sectional anatomical appearance is consistent with a loop of large bowel and its attached mesentery.
2. Diaphragmatic hernia of Morgagni type.

A diaphragmatic hernia is most commonly the result of herniation of abdominal contents through the oesophageal hiatus, a so-called hiatus hernia. It may also have a congenital or traumatic aetiology. Those secondary to trauma usually follow severe blunt abdominal injury such as may complicate a road traffic accident or a fall from a considerable height. The resulting diaphragmatic rupture generally produces a large hernia and associated respiratory distress, necessitating urgent surgical intervention. In the present case, the absence of respiratory symptoms or significant chest or abdominal injury and the history of relatively minor trauma suggests that the patient's fall was of no relevance to the radiographic abnormality. The chest film merely brought to light a pre-existing asymptomatic anterior mediastinal mass.

Congenital diaphragmatic hernias may result from herniation through the anteriorly situated foramen of Morgagni (between the costal and sternal insertions of the diaphragm) or through either of the two postero-lateral foramina of Bochdalek (the pleuroperitoneal hiatus). The latter variety may result in a large hernia filling an entire hemithorax, when the chest X-ray appearances resemble those of a large hydro-pneumothorax and clinical presentation is in the neonate with severe respiratory embarrassment. By contrast hernias through the foramen of Morgagni are generally relatively small and rarely produce symptoms. While small diaphragmatic defects may be left untreated larger defects, even those that are asymptomatic, should be considered for surgical repair as they are likely to increase in size over a period of years, especially in association with pregnancy or marked weight gain.

Table A40.1 Causes of anterior mediastinal shadows (After Simon, 1984)

Relative position of shadow	Cause
Lying in a high position	Retrosternal thyroid Aneurysmal or tortuous innominate artery Postoperative haematoma e.g. after thymectomy, cardiac surgery
Lying in the upper three-quarters of anterior mediastinum	Lymphoproliferative disorders Non-malignant mediastinal lymphadenopathy Mediastinal abscess Dermoid cyst/teratoma Cystic hygroma Thymic cyst/tumour Secondary tumour deposits Ectopic thyroid Ectopic parathyroid Lipoma/other rare benign tumours
Lying in a low position, touching diaphragm	Pleural/pericardial cyst Morgagni hernia Pericardial fat pad

The mediastinum may be arbitrarily divided into four compartments: the superior compartment extending from the thoracic inlet above to a horizontal line drawn from the fifth thoracic vertebra to the manubrio-sternal joint below; the anterior compartment lying anterior to the heart. The posterior compartment extending from the posterior aspect of the heart to the vertebrae and ribs; and the middle compartment occupied principally by the heart, great vessels and major bronchi. The lateral view radiograph makes it possible to say in which compartment a mediastinal lesion is located and, because certain lesions are characteristic of only one particular compartment, it is possible to prepare a short list of diagnostic possibilities on anatomical grounds.

Table A40.1 lists the causes of anterior mediastinal lesions according to their typical relative position. A Morgagni hernia enters the differential diagnosis of those lesions lying low in the anterior mediastinum, touching the diaphragm. When gas shadows are not seen in the plain radiograph the appearances are similar to fat pads and pleuropericardial cysts. Differentiation may be possible using barium studies or, when the hernia contains liver, by hepatic ultrasound or isotope scan. The nature of the mass is most readily identified by CT which defines the cross-sectional

180

anatomy and provides a useful measurement of tissue density (attenuation coefficient) which, in turn, will distinguish fluid-containing cysts of 'water density' from less dense lesions composed of fat.

Further reading

SIMON, G. (1984) *Principles of Chest X-ray Diagnosis.* Butterworths. London.

Case 41

Answers

1. Primary pulmonary hypertension.
2. The ECG abnormalities are: sinus tachycardia, P pulmonale, right axis deviation, right ventricular hypertrophy.
3. The overall prognosis is poor with a 10 year survival of only 25%.

Primary pulmonary hypertension is a rare but important disease which affects young people, typically women aged between 20 and 30 years (F:M ratio about 5:1). The aetiology is unknown but it may complicate clinical conditions associated with a thrombotic tendency (e.g. lupus anticoagulant) possibly by interfering with prostacyclin formation. Certain inherited thrombotic disorders (e.g. antithrombin III deficiency) may account for some of the familial cases of primary pulmonary hypertension and also for some of the cases that have developed in patients taking the anorectic drugs aminorex fumarate and fenfluramine.

The clinical diagnosis is often delayed, right heart failure being a late development and signs of a raised pulmonary vascular resistance being easily missed. A proportion of patients show features suggestive of collagen vascular disease, e.g. Raynaud's phenomenon but, in general, the leading symptoms – fatigue and dyspnoea – are non-specific. Exertional syncope and anginal pain are late features and reflect a low cardiac output and a poorer prognosis. Clinical signs of pulmonary hypertension (a loud, even palpable, pulmonary second heart sound) and right ventricular hypertrophy (parasternal heave) are often present but may be difficult to elicit. A third and/or a fourth heart sound and the murmurs of tricuspid or pulmonary incompetence may also be heard. Radiographic evidence of pulmonary hypertension or ECG changes reflecting right ventricular hypertrophy/strain are found in 95% of cases.

In clinical practice, pulmonary hypertension is most commonly encountered in association with underlying cardiac abnormality or chronic hypoxic lung disease. Rarely, severe pulmonary hypertension arises insidiously as a complication of recurrent pulmonary thromboembolism or pulmonary veno-occlusive disease. The term 'primary' (unexplained) pulmonary hypertension is appropriate when these other known causes have been excluded. Echocardiography and lung function testing will help to exclude primary cardiac and pulmonary disease and ventilation and perfusion lung scintigraphy will rule out proximal vessel thromboembolism. A significant proportion of patients with primary pulmonary hypertension will, however, show peripheral thrombotic lesions and differentiation from thromboembolic disease in this group is less clear cut. Such observations have led to the suggestion that the definitive diagnosis of primary pulmonary hypertension can only be made from lung biopsy material. The characteristic histological abnormality consists of so-called 'plexiform' lesions – dilated regions in the pulmonary arteries containing proliferating cells and new vascular channels with areas of fibrinoid necrosis – which are absent in pulmonary thromboembolic and veno-occlusive disease.

Right heart catheterization confirms the severity of pulmonary hypertension and provides prognostic information. The outlook is closely related to cardiac output: the lower the cardiac output the worse the prognosis. Most patients run a rapidly fatal course with the majority of patients dying within two years of diagnosis.

Treatment aims at improving cardiac output (using vasodilators) and preventing secondary thromboembolism. Anticoagulants will improve survival and in a small subgroup of patients there is a rise in cardiac output and symptomatic improvement in response to vasodilator therapy. These patients are best identified using prostacyclin which, with its short half-life, avoids the risk of prolonged systemic hypotension. Among responders clinical improvement and sustained reduction in pulmonary vascular resistance can be maintained with intravenous prostacyclin (by continuous infusion), nifedipine, diazoxide and isoprenaline. The agent of choice in these subjects, with reversible pulmonary hypertension, remains to be determined. For those with 'fixed' pulmonary hypertension who fail to respond in the short term, vasodilator therapy is unwise and may be deleterious; for these patients heart-lung transplantation may be the only option.

Further reading

FUSTER, V., STEELE, P. M., EDWARDS, W. D. *et al.* (1984) Primary pulmonary hypertension: a natural history and importance of thrombosis. *Circulation*, **70**, 580.

Case 42

Answers

1. Spontaneous pneumothorax.
2. Intercostal drainage should be secured (see below). If the clinical presentation suggests a tension pnemothorax but the patient appears to be tolerating the condition adequately, treatment should follow radiographic confirmation of the diagnosis. When a pneumothorax is under considerable tension and associated with severe cardio-respiratory distress, drainage may be necessary before a chest X-ray can be taken. In these circumstances the placement (in the second anterior interspace) of a large-bore cannula may be a life-saving manoeuvre, with subsequent control of the pneumothorax achieved following more leisurely insertion of an intercostal drain.

There is seldom any difficulty in diagnosing a pneumothorax when the classical clinical presentation – chest pain of sudden onset followed rapidly by shortness of breath – is associated with consistent physical signs in the chest, i.e. ipsilateral reduction in breath sounds, hyper-resonant percussion note, reduced tactile vocal fremitus and reduced vocal resonance. A tension pneumothorax is further characterized by signs of cardiovascular collapse and there may be a complete absence of breath sounds with asymmetrical expansion of the chest.

In practice, the clinical diagnosis is often less straightforward. Chest pain may be absent or minimal when there is pre-existing lung disease. The severity of breathlessness is variable depending upon the size of the pneumothorax and the presence or absence of previously compromised lung function: a relatively small pneumothorax will produce a disproportionate degree of dyspnoea in a patient with, for example, advanced pulmonary fibrosis or severe chronic obstructive lung disease. The typical physical signs may also be difficult to elicit when the pneumothorax is either small or loculated, when there is already asymmetrical chest pathology or when the chest is hyperinflated and breath sounds already impaired (as in emphysema and severe bronchial asthma). The diagnosis should always be considered when patients with underlying pulmonary disease develop an increase in symptoms.

The clinical features are non-specific and a variety of common intrathoracic disorders must often be considered in the differential diagnosis. These include pericarditis, pneumonia, myocardial infarction, pulmonary embolism and oesophageal rupture. Praecordial chest pain and respiratory distress may also accompany certain acute upper abdominal emergencies such as perforated peptic ulcer, cholecystitis and pancreatitis. In Mr Milligan's case, the sudden deterioration and development of asymmetrical chest signs against a background of severe chronic obstructive lung disease should suggest the correct diagnosis. Massive pulmonary embolism, a common event during the recovery from major medical illness, might present in a similar fashion but would not account for the asymmetrical chest signs and, in the presence of cardiovascular collapse, new ECG abnormalities would be expected.

The chest X-ray is nearly always diagnostic and depends upon the identification of the visceral pleural line which tends to parallel the shape of the chest wall. A small pneumothorax may be difficult to detect and, if suspected, a film should be taken in full expiration. Similar radiographic appearances are sometimes produced by artifacts e.g. skin folds, articles of clothing or oxygen tubing when the associated line shadows simulate the visceral pleural curve. In general, such line shadows do not run parallel to the chest wall over its entire length and their true nature can be in no doubt when their outline is traceable beyond the limits of the thorax. A large emphysematous bulla may also resemble a pneumothorax. With the aid of a bright light, however, some lung markings can usually be seen traversing the air space of the bulla. Bullae also have concave rather than convex inner margins. As a general rule, one should be wary of diagnosing a pneumothorax unless the edge of the lung can be confidently identified, with a clear space between it and the parietal pleura.

Management is influenced by a number of considerations, but particularly by the size of the pneumothorax, the severity of associated symptoms, the presence of underlying lung disease and whether or not the pneumothorax is 'open' and increasing in size or 'closed', when the air leak has sealed.

A tension pneumothorax always requires urgent intercostal drainage, sometimes before the diagnosis is confirmed radiographically, as described above. A shallow pneumothorax, occupying less than 20% of the affected hemithorax, is unlikely to cause symptoms in a previously healthy patient and, provided that the pneumothorax is 'closed', the subject may be safely observed with the expectation that the pneumothorax will have fully re-absorbed within 2–6 weeks. In a patient with pre-existing lung disease even a small pneumothorax may cause respiratory embarrassment, and active treatment is indicated. A deep pneumothorax (occupying more than 20% of the hemithorax) is more likely to be associated with symptoms when the choice of treatment lies between simple aspiration using a fine-bore catheter or underwater seal drainage. The latter approach is the one most commonly adopted although the simpler, less invasive procedure of aspiration often suffices.

Occasionally intercostal drainage fails to produce re-expansion of the lung. In exceptional cases with a very large air leak a second drain may be required. Alternatively the use of suction (-20 to -50 cm of water) applied to the chest drain will sometimes help. If after five days of continued intercostal drainage there is still evidence of a persistent air leak, thoracotomy will allow repair of the lung lesion and pleurodesis can be achieved (e.g. by pleural abrasion, parietal pleurectomy or insufflation with talc or kaolin).

About 95% of first episodes of spontaneous pneumothorax resolve with medical treatment, but a recurrence will be noted in as many as 20% of cases and among these patients the risk of a subsequent (third) pneumothorax jumps up to about 40–50%. It would seem reasonable therefore to offer elective surgery to all patients who suffer a second pneumothorax, especially if there is any likelihood of frequent travel by air or to remote places. Patients with a history of bilateral pneumothorax are at particularly high risk of recurrences (about 50% for either side) and should be offered surgery when the second lung becomes affected because of the slight but significant risk of simultaneous bilateral pneumothoraces.

Further reading

HARVEY, J. E. and JEYASINGHAM, K. (1987) The difficult pneumothorax. *British Journal of Diseases of the Chest*, **81**, 209.

Case 43

Answers

1. Extrinsic allergic alveolitis due to avian protein hypersensitivity (bird fancier's lung, pigeon breeder's disease).
2. Estimation of serum precipitating antibody to avian antigens. Lung biopsy might also be of diagnostic value but this would be hazardous in the presence of severe hypoxaemia.

The typical clinical features of extrinsic allergic alveolitis have already been described in connection with farmer's lung (see Answer 39). In bird fancier's lung too the clinical features vary depending upon the periodicity, duration and intensity of exposure. Among budgerigar fanciers antigen exposure tends to be of a low intensity and continuous rather than intermittent. In these circumstances an acute presentation is unusual. Symptoms develop insidiously and patients usually present with chronic cough, progressive breathlessness and weight loss and they will often show radiographic evidence of established pulmonary fibrosis.

An acute presentation is more characteristic of pigeon fanciers among whom antigen exposure is typically heavy and intermittent. The diagnosis readily springs to mind when the acute illness (malaise, fever, myalgia, dry cough, breathlessness) follows a clear history of relevant exposure after an interval of 6–8 hours – the classical picture. On occasion, however, there may be no clear cut temporal relationship between exposure and symptoms. This is especially the case when the illness follows 'bystander' exposure and when the presentation is subacute as was the case with Mrs Finney. Although alveolitis is usually associated with heavy antigen exposure there is variation in susceptibility and, once sensitized, some individuals may develop clinical illness in association with relatively low levels of exposure.

Mrs Finney's general practitioner, perhaps not surprisingly, had failed to appreciate the importance of the limited contact that she had had with her husband's pigeons. Certainly, many of the features of acute or subacute allergic alveolitis may be reproduced by influenza, viral pneumonia, miliary tuberculosis or sarcoidosis. Even on clinical grounds, however, none of these diagnoses adequately accounts for all of the features in Mrs Finney's case and she was started on steroids for a presumptive diagnosis of allergic alveolitis before the result of serum avian precipitins became available.

Both sarcoidosis and miliary tuberculosis may present subacutely and both conditions produce diffuse, bilateral nodular radiographic shadowing. However, neither condition, even when there is extensive pulmonary infiltration, typically produces the degree of breathlessness or such marked impairment of gas exchange as was shown by Mrs Finney. Indeed, respiratory symptoms and functional changes are characteristically mild in relation to the disproportionately severe radiographic changes. Furthermore, patients with sarcoidosis are usually in good health and without systemic symptoms. Constitutional upset is generally marked in patients with miliary tuberculosis but a negative tuberculin test, although it can occur, provides further strong evidence against this diagnosis.

Viral bronchopneumonia or 'atypical pneumonia' (e.g. psittacosis, Q fever, mycoplasma pneumonia) clearly must also be considered in the differential diagnosis. The radiographic findings are not inconsistent and severe infection may progress to respiratory failure. Fulminant pulmonary infection would be expected to pursue a more rapid course than was the case with Mrs Finney's illness. Whereas breathlessness is a feature of severe pneumonias, it occurs late in the course of the illness in a deteriorating patient and generally not as a presenting symptom (pneumonia due to Pneumocystis carinii is an exception). The duration of Mrs Finney's illness, therefore, and her initial complaint of breathlessness render viral and 'atypical' infection rather unlikely. This conclusion is supported by the results of viral titres. Normally only paired sera (acute and convalescent samples) would be tested, but with a 3 week history of symptoms an abnormal result will sometimes be obtained on the first sample; the absence of any significant titres makes unlikely, but does not completely exclude, the specific infections for which tests were carried out. Some care is required when interpreting raised viral titres; the generalized hyperglobulinaemia of allergic alveolitis may produce raised antibody titres to a variety of viral antigens (an anamnestic response), when there is the danger of incorrectly diagnosing a viral illness. About 25% of patients with acute allergic alveolitis will also have low titres of circulating rheumatoid and antinuclear factors for the same reason.

Mrs Finney's pulmonary function tests showed the expected changes with restriction of lung volumes and impaired gas transfer. The observed neutrophil leucocytosis and raised ESR are also fully consistent with an acute or subacute presentation of allergic alveolitis. The diagnosis was confirmed by the finding of a high titre of serum precipitating antibody to avian antigen. About 40% of asymptomatic pigeon breeders have demonstrable serum antibody. Therefore their presence does not necessarily signify disease. When placed in the context of Mrs Finney's clinical illness, however, positive precipitins leave little doubt about the diagnosis. Lung biopsy in acute/subacute allergic alveolitis will often show diagnostic changes but this is seldom necessary. The characteristic pathological appearance consists of non-caseating 'sarcoid-like' epithelioid and giant cell granulomata in the alveolar walls and around respiratory bronchioles along with a variable and sometimes extensive non-granulomatous infiltrate of polymorphs, lymphocytes and plasma cells. The accumualation of 'foam cells' – large histiocytes with pale vacuolated cytoplasm – is particularly characteristic of pigeon breeder's disease.

Case 44

Answers

1. Progressive systemic sclerosis.
2. Treatment is symptomatic. No therapy has been shown convincingly to alter the the course of the disease.
3. The prognosis is determined by the extent of visceral involvement and is particularly poor in patients with clinical evidence of renal, cardiac or pulmonary disease. The outcome in patients with pulmonary involvement is similar to that in patients with cryptogenic fibrosing alveolitis – about 50% die within five years of diagnosis.

The clinical picture of fibrosing alveolitis may occur in isolation (see Answer 21) or in association with a variety of 'connective tissue disorders' (Table A44.1). These disorders present overlapping patterns of clinical and immunological abnormality and are characterized by the presence of organ specific autoantibodies (e.g. thyroid disease, pernicious anaemia), non-organ-specific autoantibodies (e.g. rheumatoid disease, systemic sclerosis, SLE), both types of autoantibody (e.g. Sjögren's syndrome) or neither type (e.g. polymyositis, dermatomyositis). Usually the combined clinical and immunological features suggest a precise diagnosis. Occasionally the overall picture is such a 'hybrid' as to justify the clinical description 'overlap syndrome'.

Table A44.1   Connective tissue disorders associated with fibrosing alveolitis

Rheumatoid arthritis
Progressive systemic sclerosis
Systemic lupus erythematosus
Mixed connective tissue disease
Sjögren's syndrome
Polymyositis/dermatomyositis
Chronic active hepatitis
Renal tubular acidosis
Ulcerative colitis
Autoimmune thyroid disease
Pernicious anaemia

Lung involvement in systemic sclerosis runs a similar course to that of 'lone' fibrosing alveolitis. However, the combination of sclerodermatous skin changes, pulmonary fibrosis and radiological abnormalities of the oesophagus is virtually diagnostic of progressive systemic sclerosis. This is a multisystem disease characterized by varying degrees of inflammation, atrophy and fibrosis in affected organs. The peak age incidence is in the fifth decade and females are more commonly affected than males in a ratio of 3:1.

Lung involvement is common and is evident at postmortem in about 90% of affected patients. During life about 25% of subjects show overt radiographic abnormalities, but a far larger proportion will show abnormalities on pulmonary function testing (restrictive ventilatory defect, increased lung compliance and impaired gas transfer). There is commonly a coexisting pulmonary vasculitis and occasionally, when this is the predominant lesion, the clinical picture is that of progressive pulmonary hypertension. Rarely, severe pulmonary hypertension arises in the absence of either radiological or functional evidence of alveolitis. In these circumstances, clinical signs of multisystem involvement and immunological abnormality (hyperglobulinaemia, positive antinuclear antibodies in 50–70% of patients) serve to differentiate from 'primary' and thromboembolic causes of pulmonary hypertension. In some cases dyspnoea may also result from respiratory muscle weakness secondary to chest wall and/or diaphragmatic involvement when, in the absence of significant pulmonary fibrosis, extrapulmonary restriction with normal gas transfer would be expected on physiological testing. Pulmonary involvement in systemic sclerosis, as in cryptogenic fibrosing alveolitis, is associated with an increased death rate from lung cancer which is some ten times that of a control population.

Oesophageal involvement is found in about 50% of patients. Oesophageal dilatation, reduced peristalsis and reduction in the lower oesophageal sphincter pressure are the characteristic features. Symptomatic oesophagitis is common and is occasionally severe enough to result in oesophageal stricture and associated pulmonary complications due to 'overspill pneumonitis'. Oesophageal changes invariably constitute the first manifestation of gastro-intestinal involvement. Other gastro-intestinal manifestations include prolonged transit time, colonic saccular diverticulae, and duodenal dilatation with bacterial overgrowth and secondary malabsorption.

After skin, pulmonary and gastro-intestinal involvement the other major clinical manifestations relate to musculoskeletal, cardiac and renal changes. Survival is closely related to the degree and type of visceral involvement, increasingly adverse effects on prognosis being associated with pulmonary, cardiac and especially renal disease. Treatment is largely symptomatic and is directed towards the specific organ systems affected. Although the pulmonary fibrosis of systemic sclerosis is preceded by an alveolitis, there is no convincing evidence that treatment with corticosteroids or immunosuppressant therapy alters the course of the disease.

Further reading

HUNNINGHAKE, G. W. and FAUCI, A. S. (1979) Pulmonary involvement in the collagen vascular diseases. *American Review of Respiratory Diseases,* **119,** 471.

Case 45

Answers

1 Assisted ventilation.
2 (a) At each stage prior to his hospital admission there was a lack of objective assessment. Peak flow monitoring by the general practitioner or by the patient may well have indicated the need for additional anti-asthmatic therapy well in advance of his admission to hospital.
(b) Mr Clements was slow to seek further advice when he was clearly getting worse. Asthmatics need to be educated as to how and when they must respond when they deteriorate.
(c) The 'emergency doctor' failed to recognize the severity of Mr Clements' attack of asthma. Treatment with steroids should have been initiated and hospital admission arranged at this stage.
(d) Intravenously administered bronchodilators may increase hypoxaemia in acute severe asthma and they should be used in conjunction with oxygen therapy.
(e) Severe hypoxaemia in acute asthma should be treated with high-dose oxygen (FiO_2, 40–60%) and not controlled (24–28%) oxygen.

Regrettably, asthma is often mismanaged by both primary care physicians and hospital doctors alike. Errors of clinical judgment such as those described above occur all too frequently and these may contribute to mortality: each year, there are about 1500 deaths from this cause in England and Wales. Retrospective studies of asthma deaths both at home and in hospital show that they commonly occur at night and are often unexpected. They may occur with overwhelming suddeness before medical attention can be summoned. More commonly deterioration occurs over a period of days or weeks. In both instances, however, it is often possible to identify serious inadequacies in prior management.

A recurring feature of both hospital and community-based studies has been the underuse of corticosteroid drugs and inadequate objective assessment of asthma severity. The patients themselves may fail to appreciate the gravity of their condition: the perception of breathlessness among asthmatics is very variable and some, particularly those with persistent symptoms and those with frequent acute asthma, acquire a degree of tolerance

Table A45.1   Clinical grading of asthma severity (from Jones, 1971)

Grade	Severity of asthma
1A	Patient able to carry out housework or job with moderate difficulty; sleep occasionally disturbed
1B	Patient only able to carry out housework or job with great difficulty; sleep frequently disturbed.
2A	Patient confined to chair or bed but able to get up with moderate difficulty; sleep disturbed with little or no relief from inhaler.
2B	Patient confined to chair or bed and only able to get up with great difficulty; unable to sleep; pulse rate over 120 beats/min.
3	Patient totally confined to chair or bed; no sleep; no relief from inhaler; pulse rate over 120 beats/min.
4	Patient moribund.

(temporal adaptation) and as a consequence they may be slow to take remedial action during an attack. In a study of asthma deaths in two regions of England (Research Committee of the British Thoracic Association, 1982), supervision by general practitioners leading up to the fatal attack was considered adequate in only 2 out of the 90 asthmatics. Failure of both patient and doctor to appreciate the severity of the attack, inadequate therapy (with bronchodilators and corticosteroids), delay in seeing the patient at home and delay in transferring the patient to hospital all occurred commonly.

Successful management of bronchial asthma is clearly dependent upon an accurate assessment of its clinical severity. A variety of schemes have been used to grade severity, perhaps the best known being that devised by Jones (1971). This basically provides an index of loss of exercise tolerance (Table A45.1). Jones recommended hospital admission when the patient reached grade 2A. A PEFR of 150 l/min or less should also alert the doctor to the possible need for hospital admission. Some clinical features are more reliable indicators of asthma severity (Table A45.2) than others. Wheeze is an almost invariable feature of acute asthma but its absence may, paradoxically, suggest a particularly severe attack when airflow is too low to generate wheeze. Cyanosis is a feature of life-threatening asthma but its detection is liable to subjective error. Measurement of arterial blood gases is mandatory when the PEFR is less than 100 l/min.

Assisted ventilation can be life-saving but is rarely necessary in the management of acute severe asthma, the vast majority of patients responding to conventional combined treatment using a

192

Table A45.2	Clinical criteria of severe acute asthma

Loss of exercise tolerance (2A or worse in Jones' classification)
$PEFR < 100\,l/min$
Pulse rate > 120 beats/min
Palpable pulsus paradoxus
ECG abnormalities
Gross radiographic evidence of hyperinflation
Severe hypoxaemia (central cyanosis; arterial $Pao_2 < 7.98\,kPa$
CO_2 retention ($Paco_2 > 5.98\,kPa$), and especially a rising $Paco_2$
Obvious exhaustion
Impairment of consciousness

nebulized β_2 agonist, parenteral steroids and oxygen, with or without the additional use of nebulized ipratropium and parenteral aminophylline. The need for mechanical ventilation arises in association with cardiorespiratory arrest or, more commonly, when the patient deteriorates despite intensive medical therapy. In this latter group ventilation is usually initiated in response to signs of exhaustion in a patient who may also show worsening hypoxaemia, a climbing pulse and/or respiratory rate and a falling PEFR. An elevated $Paco_2$ points to a severe attack of asthma but is not in itself an indication for mechanical ventilation. Trends in arterial blood gases are of greater importance. A rising $Paco_2$ in an exhausted patient is a particularly ominous sign and will usually suggest the need for ventilatory support.

References

JONES, E. S. (1971) The intensive therapy of asthma. Proceedings of the Royal Society of Medicine, **64**, 1151.
RESEARCH COMMITTEE OF THE BRITISH THORACIC ASSOCIATION (1982) Death from asthma in two regions of England. British Medical Journal, **285**, 1251.

Case 46

Answers

1. Legionnaire's disease
2. Erythromycin is the antibiotic of choice. In very sick patients intravenous rifampicin should also be given.

The hospital diagnosis of pneumonia presents little difficulty when there is a history of an acute febrile illness associated with respiratory symptoms and 'fresh' radiographic shadowing. When there are prominent extrathoracic manifestations, acute presentations of systemic vasculitis or metastatic bronchial carcinoma (with secondary pulmonary infection) are a potential source of confusion. In practice, the greater problem lies not with the diagnosis of pneumonia, but with the assessment of its specific microbiological cause. Reference has already been made to the limited range of pathogens that are most commonly implicated in community-acquired pneumonia (see Answer 22). In general, their presentations are not sufficiently distinctive to allow confident clinical diagnosis. However, the spectrum of clinical/biochemical abnormalities and certain other features (e.g. history of recent foreign travel – legionella infection; contact with farm animals – Q fever; recent influenza – staphylococcal pneumonia; contact with birds – psittacosis) will sometimes raise clinical suspicion to a level which may assist in early clinical management.

Legionnaire's disease is the pneumonia caused by the gram-negative bacillus, *Legionella pneumophila* of which ten serotypes have been identified. This and other *Legionella* species are ubiquitous in nature and grow best in warm stagnant water. Respiratory infection is by the inhaled route with an incubation period of 2–10 days. Sporadic cases show marked geographical variation and account for about 1.5–15% of community-acquired pneumonias in the UK. Epidemic infection is closely associated with contaminated water systems (air-conditioning systems, shower units, cooling towers) and is most often encountered in relation to large buildings e.g. hotels and hospitals. Certain host factors influence the likelihood of infection: it is unusual in children and typically affects the middle-aged or elderly. Male sex (M:F ratio, 3:1), heavy smoking habit, heavy alcohol consumption, underlying chronic cardiopulmonary disease, chronic renal failure, diabetes mellitus and immunosuppressive therapy have all been identified as risk factors.

There is a wide spectrum of clinical illness ranging from asymptomatic sero-conversion and mild non-pneumonic illness (Pontiac fever) to severe pneumonia with or without extrapulmonary manifestations. The mortality rate in published series ranges from 10–15%. The onset is usually over several days with a prodrome of malaise, anorexia, lethargy, headache and myalgia. Preceding upper respiratory symptoms are usually absent. The illness evolves with cough, usually non-productive, febrile symptoms and dyspnoea. Haemoptysis and pleuritic pain each occurs in about a third of patients. Watery diarrhoea occurs in about half of the cases. CNS abnormalities are encountered in about 25% of patients, confusion and disorientation being the most common features. Hallucinations, generalized seizures, cerebellar dysfunction and peripheral neuropathy have all been described.

The patient usually appears acutely ill. Fever is almost invariable and reaches 40°C or above in about half of the cases. Relative bradycardia is common (two-thirds of cases) and tachypnoea is present in proportion to the extent of the pneumonia. Clinical findings in the chest are often limited to crackles in the early stages, but signs of consolidation subsequently appear in the majority of patients. The radiographic picture is non-specific, i.e. patchy alveolar consolidation which is usually (70% of cases) confined to a single lobe. Small pleural effusions are seen occasionally and, rarely, cavitation occurs as a late feature in areas of consolidated lung. Complete radiographic resolution may be delayed for several months.

Laboratory investigations frequently reveal a range of abnormalities which, although non-specific in themselves, point to a multisystem disorder and, when placed in the clinical context, may help to diagnose *Legionella* infection as opposed to other causes of pneumonia. Urinalysis commonly shows haematuria, proteinuria and, rarely, myoglobinuria. Hyponatraemia, hypophosphataemia, raised levels of serum creatine phosphokinase, hepatic transaminases, alkaline phosphatase and bilirubin have all been frequently noted. There is usually a modest elevation in the total white blood cell count with a neutrophil leucocytosis and, commonly, an absolute lymphopenia ($< 1 \times 10^9$/l).

Legionella pneumophila may be cultured from respiratory secretions using special techniques, but these are not applied in most routine laboratories. Diagnostic confirmation is usually made retrospectively as the result of a fourfold rise in titre in the indirect fluorescent antibody test. The test is highly specific but sero-conversion does not occur in about 10–20% of patients. Tests based on direct immunofluoresence of respiratory secretions and urine, offer the possibility of rapid diagnosis; they are highly specific but only moderately sensitive and are not in routine use. Until such tests are more widely available, the choice of initial antibiotic therapy in community-acquired pneumonia must remain largely empirical. Only occasionally, as with Mr Lennox, are the combined clinical and laboratory features sufficiently distinctive to reliably suggest the correct diagnosis.

Further reading

EDELSTEIN, P. H. and MEYER, R. D. (1984) Legionnaire's disease. A review. *Chest*, **85**, 114.

WOODHEAD, M. A. and MacFARLANE, J. T. (1987) Comparative clinical and laboratory features of legionella with pneumococcal and mycoplasma pneumonias. *British Journal of Diseases of the Chest*, **81**, 133.

Case 47

Answers

1. There is a severe, irreversible obstructive ventilatory defect with air trapping and impaired gas transfer. The total lung capacity is inappropriately normal relative to the degree of airflow obstruction suggesting the possibility of additional, 'restriction' i.e. a combined obstructive and restrictive ventilatory defect.
2. Coalworkers's pneumoconiosis complicated by progressive massive fibrosis (PMF).

'Simple' coalworker's pneumoconiosis (CWP) is characterized radiographically by the presence of multiple small rounded opacities which are distributed diffusely throughout both lung fields, i.e. changes fully consistent with Mr McCulloch's X-ray report upon his retirement. 'Simple' CWP is not, however, associated with clinically significant impairment of lung function. As a group, coalminers show a slightly lower mean FEV_1 than comparable control subjects. However, for patients with 'simple' CWP spirometric abnormalities are related primarily to the effects of smoking cigarettes rather than to the effects of coal dust. Clearly, therefore, Mr McCulloch's breathlessness at this stage must be attributed to some other aetiology – almost certainly chronic obstructive lung disease – although alternative causes of diffuse radiographic shadowing (e.g. sarcoidosis, 'early' fibrosing alveolitis) must come into the differential diagnosis.

When he presented, some nine years after his retirement, breathlessness has progressed and the radiographic picture had changed, with the appearance of bilateral well-defined areas of homogeneous shadowing in both upper zones. The predominantly obstructive defect of ventilation and associated features (wheeze, signs of hyperinflation) of airflow obstruction render sarcoidosis and fibrosing alveolitis highly improbable on clinical grounds. Pulmonary metastases complicating previously resected colonic carcinoma are an unlikely cause of such symmetrical mass lesions, especially in the absence of other evidence of metastatic disease. The radiographic appearances are, however, characteristic of progressive massive fibrosis (PMF). 'Simple' CWP rarely either progresses or regresses after dust exposure has ceased. However, PMF may develop for the first time long after the patient has left the industry, as was the case here.

The lesions of PMF produce rounded or oval homogeneous shadows, having an arbitrary diameter greater than 1 cm. They may be unilateral but are usually bilateral and most often affect the upper lobes. In the early stages the lesions tend to be irregular and ill-defined. They characteristically increase in size over a period of years, become better defined and tend to migrate towards the hilum leaving an area of emphysematous lung peripherally. There is usually background nodular shadowing due to 'simple' pneumoconiosis and when there is related occupational exposure there can be little doubt about the diagnosis. Mr McCulloch's extensive weight loss might appear to suggest more sinister pathology: bronchial carcinoma may resemble a unilateral mass lesion of PMF and either unilateral or bilateral upper zone PMF may mimic tuberculosis. However, weight loss is also a common feature of progressive respiratory disability, particularly among overtly emphysematous patients, and its gradual development (over 2–3 years) in this patient is more in keeping with this cause rather than any infective or neoplastic complication.

The functional abnormalities in PMF are variable and depend upon the size and site of the fibrotic lesions, as well as the presence or absence of 'scar' or 'panlobular' emphysema and chronic obstructive bronchitis. The usual finding is a predominantly obstructive ventilatory defect but the presence of mixed pathology commonly results in the pattern seen here: airflow obstruction (low FEV_1/FVC ratio) with a reduced VC and a raised RV, but with a normal TLC. This is the net result of opposite influences, airflow obstruction producing hyperinflation and fibrosis producing some shrinkage in total lung volume.

The greater the degree of exposure to coal dust the greater the risk of developing 'simple' CWP and that this will subsequently progress to PMF. Men at risk are offered periodic X-rays and those found to have radiographic evidence of 'simple' disease are given appropriate medical advice. The industry is also legally required to offer alternative work where dust levels are known to be low and to provide further medical supervision. With improved methods of underground ventilation and dust control over the last two decades, there has in fact been a progressive decline in the number of certifications of CWP and, currently, most new cases (about 400 per year) are diagnosed among ex-miners like Mr McCulloch. Affected patients should be advised to apply for industrial disablement benefit. There is no effective treatment for established pneumoconiosis and any active measures relate only to the management of complications (respiratory infection, cor pulmonale).

Case 48

Answers

1. Acute massive pulmonary embolism.
2. Thrombolytic therapy (e.g. streptokinase, urokinase).

The clinical presentation of pulmonary embolism is dependent upon the size and number of emboli, the patient's previous cardiopulmonary status, the rate at which clot fragmentation and lysis occurs and upon whether or not there is a source from which recurrent embolism may occur. Three fairly distinct clinical pictures may be seen: pulmonary infarction, thromboembolic pulmonary hypertension and acute massive pulmonary embolism, defined angiographically as 50% or greater obstruction of the pulmonary arterial bed. A wide variety of circumstances predispose to thromboembolic disease (Table A48.1) and in individual cases, as with Mrs Warren (obesity, immobilization, cardiac disease, underlying malignancy), it is common to find that a number of risk factors apply.

Her presentation is typical of acute massive pulmonary embolism. The clinical diagnosis is supported by ECG evidence of right heart strain (right axis deviation, 'acute' right bundle branch block, T wave inversion in the right chest leads – V1–V4); the classical $S_1Q_3T_3$ pattern is rare and, commonly, a sinus tachycardia is the only ECG abnormality. The plain chest X-ray may show peripheral segmental shadows or other abnormalites (linear atelectasis, raised hemidiaphragm) resulting from a previous embolic episode. The lung fields may show areas of increased translucency caused by a paucity of vessels and indicating areas of oligaemia. The hilar shadows may appear plump due to a combination of clot within the artery and distension by the raised pulmonary artery pressure proximal to the thrombus. Often, however, the chest X-ray shows no abnormality. In addition to the features seen here the patient commonly complains of central chest pain due to reduced coronary blood flow and associated myocardial ischaemia such that acute myocardial infarction and aortic dissection must be considered in the differential diagnosis. Circulatory failure associated with a tension pneumothorax is readily differentiated by careful physical examination and by the appearances of the chest film. Adventitious sounds are normally absent in massive pulmonary embolism but, occasionally, there is generalized wheeze with the potential for misdiagnosing acute asthma which may also be associated with ECG evidence of right heart strain. Definitive confirmation of the diagnosis may be obtained by ventilation and perfusion lung scintigraphy or by pulmonary angiography. In practice, however, treatment for acute massive pulmonary embolism must frequently be instituted before confirmatory diagnostic investigations can be arranged and, more

Table A48.1   Risk factors for thromboembolic disease

Recent surgery	Miscellaneous disorders
Trauma	Cushing's syndrome
Pre-existing cardiopulmonary disease	Behçet's syndrome
Previous history of thromboembolic disease	Ulcerative colitis
	Homocystinuria
Family history of thromboembolic disease	Immobilization
	Obesity
Oral contraceptive/oestrogen therapy	Underlying malignancy
Myeloproliferative disorders	Pregnancy/puerperium
Certain coagulation disorders, e.g.	Blood group A
Antithrombin 3 deficiency	Gram-negative sepsis
Lupus anticoagulant	

often than not, the initial choice of therapy must be based upon clinical considerations.

Heparin anticoagulation represents inadequate treatment for patients with considerable haemodynamic embarrassment. Where massive pulmonary embolism is associated with sustained arterial hypotension (systolic blood pressure of 100 mmHg or less), severe hypoxia, poor peripheral perfusion and reduced urine flow, thrombolytic therapy is indicated. It is often said that pulmonary angiography is mandatory prior to the initiation of thrombolytic treatment because of the risks inherent in this approach. In fact comparative studies have shown that the risk of serious haemorrhage is approximately the same (7%) for both heparin and thrombolytic drugs. Furthermore, most episodes of massive embolism occur in hospitals without the facilities for angiography and transfer to a centre with such facilities is hardly appropriate in this group of critically ill patients. Using pulmonary angiography as the gold standard the clinical diagnosis of pulmonary embolism is inaccurate in over 50% of patients suspected of having pulmonary embolism. However, diagnostic errors are most frequent among patients with smaller emboli for whom thrombolytic therapy would not be used; with massive pulmonary embolism clinical diagnostic certainty (with or without lung scanning) is usually sufficiently strong to allow thrombolytic therapy without the need for prior angiography. When thrombolytic therapy is contraindicated pulmonary embolectomy should be undertaken.

There is a high early death rate associated with acute massive pulmonary embolism. There is also a high late mortality rate (15–30%) among patients who survive to leave hospital, most deaths being due to other underlying disease (especially cardiopulmonary disease and malignancy) rather than recurrent pulmonary emboli. Mrs Warren survived her episode of pulmonary embolism only to succumb six months later from a high grade malignant lymphoma which responded poorly to treatment.

Further reading

BENATAR, S. R., IMMELMAN, E. J. and JEFFREY, P. (1986) Pulmonary embolism. *British Journal of Diseases of the Chest*, **80**, 313.

EDITORIAL (1985) Difficulties in the treatment of acute pulmonary embolism. *Thorax*, **40**, 729.

Case 49

Answers

1. Systemic lupus erythematosus.
2. (a) Enlargement of the cardiac silhouette is probably the result of a pericardial effusion.
   (b) Elevation of both leaves of the diaphragm could merely reflect a poor inspiratory effort. The restrictive defect of lung function suggests that this is not the explanation, but that this represents the 'shrinking lung syndrome' due to a localized myositis affecting the diaphragm (see below).

The collagen vascular diseases are a heterogeneous group of disorders of unknown aetiology and uncertain pathogenesis. The conditions tend to share the same range of clinical manifestations (inflammation of joints, serosal membranes, connective tissues and blood vessels in a variety of organs) but a number of well defined clinical syndromes may be recognized. Among these, the lungs, with their abundant vasculature and extensive framework of connective tissue, are a common site of disease involvement. The lungs and pleura are capable of responding to injury in only a limited number of ways and the various clinical syndromes therefore show similar patterns of abnormality. In some cases, however, a more distinctive pattern of lung involvement is seen which may aid clinical diagnosis. The typical pleuropulmonary manifestations of systemic sclerosis (Answer 44), rheumatoid disease (Answer 28) and systemic vasculitis (Answer 32) have already been discussed. Those associated with systemic lupus erythematosus (SLE) are summarized in Table A49.1.

Table A49.1 **Pleuropulmonary complications of systemic lupus erythematosus**

Pleurisy with or without effusion
Diffuse interstitial pneumonitis
Diaphragmatic myopathy
Basal atelectasis
Acute 'lupus' pneumonitis (pulmonary vasculitis, haemorrhage)
Increased frequency of respiratory infection
Pulmonary hypertension (rare)

SLE is characteristically a disease of young women (F:M ratio, 10:1) in their second or third decade. Its variable course is punctuated by episodes of disease activity which often remit postmenopausally. There is a strong association with a wide variety of non organ-specific autoantibodies and the demonstration of serum antinuclear antibodies (ANF) offers a reliable screening test for SLE in the appropriate clinical setting. The presence of antibodies to double-stranded DNA offers a more specific diagnostic test which, in some patients, may also reflect disease activity. The clinical manifestations are legion. Non-specific features such as malaise, lethargy, depression and fever commonly dominate the course of the disease. Among the more specific features musculoskeletal and cutaneous involvement are the most frequent. Arthralgia or non-erosive polyarthritis, often in rheumatoid distribution, occurs in about 85% of patients and, along with the various skin lesions ('butterfly' rash, vasculitic rashes, livedo reticularis, alopecia, discoid rashes, photosensitivity and Raynaud's phenomenon), constitutes the most common clinical presentation. In contrast to rheumatoid arthritis, glomerulonephritis is common (40–75%) and, together with CNS involvement (psychosis, seizures, cerebral thrombosis, transverse myelitis), is a major determinant of survival. Among the many other extrapulmonary manifestations are: pericarditis, myocarditis, endocarditis, myalgia, myositis, haematological abnormalities (anaemia, leucopenia, thrombocytopenia), oral/nasal ulcers, venous thrombosis, recurrent abortion and false positive serological tests for syphilis.

Pleuritis, with or without effusion, occurs at some stage in as many as 50–75% of patients and may be the presenting abnormality. Episodes of pleuritic pain typically last several days. They may be unilateral or bilateral and are commonly accompanied by fever and evidence of pericarditis which was the predominant feature of Mrs Stephens' presentation. The effusions are small or moderate in size and otherwise similar to those complicating rheumatoid disease (a straw-coloured exudate with a predominant mononuclear cell content) except for the occasional presence of LE cells and pleural fluid glucose concentrations which tend to be less markedly depressed. A predominance of polymorphs should suggest the possibility of bacterial infection.

Diffuse interstitial pulmonary fibrosis is less common in SLE than in other collagen diseases. One series showed a frequency of only 3%, while several large series have failed to record any cases at all. As with fibrosing alveolitis due to other causes only a proportion of patients respond favourably to corticosteroids. A more distinctive abnormality is occasionally seen when elevated diaphragms, which move 'sluggishly' on screening, are associated with dyspnoea, orthopnoea and a restrictive ventilatory defect: the 'shrinking lung syndrome'. Affected patients generally show a reduction in total gas transfer capacity and decreased maximum transdiaphragmatic pressure. Most patients give a past history of pleurisy and, formerly, the abnormalities were attributed to pleural adhesions or atelectasis. It is now believed that the primary defect is a myopathy or myositis affecting the diaphragm and that atelectasis is probably a secondary effect which merely serves to increase the functional abnormality. Orthopnoea is a typical feature of diaphragmatic weakness (see Answer 26) although, in the case of Mrs Stephens, her pericardial effusion may have contributed to this symptom. Lung volumes have been seen to increase as disease activity wanes and then remain stable for long periods, so that diaphragmatic function is clearly recoverable.

The term acute 'lupus' pneumonitis is generally applied to SLE when lung infiltrates appear rapidly in the absence of infection or pulmonary oedema. The radiological appearances are variable but most commonly consist of either unilateral or bilateral alveolar consolidation. The pathology is poorly understood, but pulmonary haemorrhage and vasculitis probably account for most cases. Patients generally respond well to corticosteroids with or without additional immunosuppressant therapy (e.g. azathioprine).

About 50% of pleuropulmonary abnormalities in SLE are secondary to infection which are an important cause of death. Patients with renal disease and those on immunosuppressant therapy are especially at risk. A high index of suspicion is required, particularly among susceptible subjects when the presence of fever and lung involvement should be regarded as infective in origin until proven otherwise.

Further reading

GIBSON, G. J., EDMONDS, J. P. and HUGHES, G. R. V. (1977) Diaphragm function and lung involvement in systemic lupus erythematosus. *American Journal of Medicine*, **63**, 926.

HUNNINGHAKE, G. W. and FAUCI, A. S. (1979) Pulmonary involvement in the collagen vascular diseases. *American Review of Respiratory Disease*, **119**, 471.

Case 50

Answers

1. Antibiotic failure was secondary to the development of a pleural empyema.
2. The main therapeutic alternatives are:
   (a) Repeated pleural aspiration with instillation of appropriate antibiotic therapy.
   (b) Closed chest drainage via an intercostal tube.
   (c) Early decortication (see below).

Despite the advent of potent antibiotics bacterial pneumonia remains an important cause of morbidity and mortality. Pneumonia is a common mode of death in elderly patients where it is often a terminal complication of a wide variety of chronic disorders. However, pneumonia is also a serious condition in younger age groups: for those under 65 years deaths due to pneumonia equal those from all other infections combined. Each year in the 5–49 year age group the death rate from pneumonia is three to four times that for bronchial asthma. Published studies over the last 25 years show an overall mortality for community-acquired pneumonia of 6–18%. Despite this most patients with uncomplicated pneumonia can be satisfactorily managed at home with hospital admission reserved for seriously ill patients, especially when tachypnoea, confusion or cyanosis is present, or when the patient fails to respond to initial antibiotic therapy.

Failure to respond to therapy after 36–48 hours should lead to reconsideration of the diagnosis and of the antibiotic policy. A similar clinical picture may be seen with pulmonary infarction and tuberculous pleural effusion, but there appears no reason in Mr Syme's case to doubt the clinical diagnosis of lobar pneumonia. Treatment with amoxycillin represents adequate first-line therapy for most community-acquired pneumonias except during influenza and mycoplasma epidemics when flucloxacillin and erythromycin, respectively, merit inclusion in the initial antibiotic regime. In the present case there were no clinical features at all suggestive of mycoplasma pneumonia, but the addition of an anti-staphylococcal antibiotic would have been a reasonable course of action when Mr Syme appeared little better after three days treatment. At the very least sputum should have been sent at this stage for bacteriological examination. Of the bacterial pathogens most likely to be associated with failure to respond to penicillin, *Mycobacterium tuberculosis* may be identifiable on direct microscopy whilst both *Staphylococcus aureus* and *Klebsiella pneumoniae* are readily cultured. A result should be available within 48 hours when appropriate adjustments in antibiotic therapy may be made. Pneumonia arising distal to a bronchial obstruction (e.g. due to bronchial carcinoma or foreign body) may also fail to respond to antibiotic therapy and if there is clinical suspicion bronchoscopy is mandatory.

In the case of Mr Syme the clinical and radiographic features strongly suggest an empyema, i.e. a purulent pleural effusion. With appropriate antibiotic therapy this is an uncommon complication, but pneumonia remains the most important underlying cause. Less commonly empyemata arise in the absence of bronchopulmonary infection (following thoracotomy, thoracocentesis, trauma, oesophageal perforation and in association with upper abdominal surgery complicated by subdiaphragmatic infection). The spectrum of bacterial pathogens depends upon the underlying aetiology. The predominant organisms in post-pneumonic empyemata are *Staphylococcus aureus* (the most important pathogen), *Streptococcus pneumoniae,* anaerobic streptococci and *Bacteroides* spp. Gram-negative enteric bacilli are the most common pathogens in empyemata following surgery.

During the course of a pneumonic illness the diagnosis of empyema is suggested by the persistence or recrudesence of respiratory symptoms and toxaemia. As the acute phase subsides pleural pain tends to resolve but a swinging fever persists with accompanying anorexia and weight loss. Finger clubbing may develop within two to three weeks. Clinical examination will usually suggest the presence of pleural fluid. The chest film shows a uniform opacity either free within the pleural space or encysted by adhesions. In the presence of much consolidation decubitus views may be useful in order to identify the amount of free pleural fluid. Most empyemata lie postero-laterally and often produce a D-shaped opacity in the lateral view radiograph. Confirmation of the diagnosis is by pleural aspiration. When pus is loculated thoracic ultrasound may be very useful for determining the best site for aspiration or drainage.

The aims of treatment are threefold: adequate drainage of the pleural collection, sterilization of the infection and obliteration of the empyema cavity so that the underlying lung can re-expand. Inadequate or delayed pleural drainage is associated with increased morbidity and mortality and the importance of the first aim of treatment cannot be over-emphasized. Repeated pleural aspiration (as opposed to closed chest drainage) has no place in the management of frankly purulent effusions. If diagnostic pleural aspiration yields very turbid material or thick pus, closed chest tube drainage should be instituted without delay. The earlier adequate drainage is instituted the greater the likelihood of success. Para-pneumonic effusions which are neither turbid nor frankly purulent will often resolve with antibiotic therapy alone, especially if they are small. Larger effusions with these characteristics may be managed by repeated pleural aspiration, but closed chest drainage is preferable.

Closed chest drainage combined with appropriate antibiotic therapy yields satisfactory results in about 60% of patients with aerobic infection and in a somewhat smaller proportion of patients with anaerobic infection. When pleural sepsis is not controlled by these means decortication is the treatment of choice. The procedure requires a formal thoracotomy when the oedematous and thickened pleura is removed and all pus is evacuated from the pleural space, allowing the underlying lung to expand. Decortication should only be considered when pleural infection is not adequately controlled. It should not be used merely to remove thickened pleura in the acute stage because this usually resolves spontaneously over a period of months. Because of the frequent failure of closed chest drainage in the management of empyema and the subsequent requirement for surgical treatment, hospital stay is often prolonged. Early decortication (in preference to closed chest drainage) has therefore found favour in some centres as a means of achieving rapid and effective control of pleural sepsis with expansion of the underlying lung and reduced hospital stay.

Further reading

LIGHT, R. W. (1983) Parapneumonic effusions and infections of the pleural space. In *Pleural Diseases*. Lea and Febiger, Philadelphia, p. 101.

Index

Note: Page numbers in *italics* refer to those pages on which the case presentation appears, but where the disorder is not named. 'vs' denotes differential diagnosis.